CU00406347

This book is for you if...

- You already have diabetes, either type 1 or type 2.
- You are pre diabetic or at heightened risk of developing it later in life.
- You have already noticed deterioration in your feet.
- You want to manage your condition rather than letting it manage you.
- You have just been diagnosed with diabetes and can't accept it – this book is here to help you regain hope for what your future can hold.
- You haven't taken your diagnosis seriously and need a wake-up call!
- You are fearful about what the future holds.
- You are feeling lonely since your diagnosis.
- You have already had an amputation and want to safeguard against further surgery.
- You feel like a failure for repeatedly giving in and eating naughty but nice things or perhaps you don't exercise as you know you should.
- Your feet are stopping you from being as active as you need or want to be.
- You have already been told your feet are at risk or you already have active diabetic foot disease.
- A loved one or friend has diabetes and you want to make a positive difference to their life.
- You have deformities in your feet, such as bunions or hammer toes, corns or calluses.
- You are a health professional, or carer, or you work in a nursing home and would like to use this book as a resource.
- You have had diabetes for some time and have become a bit complacent about it.
- You want to discover how you or your loved one can live in the safest possible way with their condition.

What people are saying about
Undefeeted...

"Every 20 seconds, somewhere in the world, an amputation is performed on a person with diabetes. The good news is that nearly all of these are ultimately avoidable. My colleagues at SALSA and I wholeheartedly support the efforts of Peter and Tina and look forward to a day when we can remain Undefeeted."

Dr. David G Armstrong
Professor of surgery, University of Arizona, USA.
Director, Southern Arizona Limb Salvage Alliance (SALSA)

"This is a very powerful book...

I loved the interactive aspects to help the reader analyze his or her current medical situation. You also make a great case on how we routinely see the dentist, but ignore the one part of our body that takes us where we need to go - our feet.

As somebody with a father and father-in-law with diabetes, I would make this essential reading. In fact, the idea of taking care of your feet, also makes this book an essential read, even if you are not diabetic."

Tom Coyle
Former Army captain, Dept of State Foreign Service Officer, and President of Adventures in Leadership

---

"Wow. Peter is really going to inspire people. It's true knowledge and awareness means nothing if you don't add the magic... taking action.

I am seeing in my consulting room people are living in denial about their diabetes.

I am fully supportive of this fantastic initiative to raise awareness and educate the masses. This book couldn't have come at a better time!"

Dr Grace Oppong
Medical practitioner, A & E, Effia Nkwanta Regional Hospital, Ghana

---

"It's very well written and easy to read, I found it absolutely amazing, quite mind-blowing and I wish there had been something like it around when I got diabetes.

The diabetic sweet spot is a great idea! I highly recommend that everyone reads this book, but most certainly if you have diabetes, you must!"

Elizabeth S.
Surrey, UK

"Any movement or crusade to reduce the number of amputations in diabetic patients needs our full praise and support, so I heartily endorse this crusade!"

Prof Mike Edmonds
Consultant Diabetologist, Kings College Hospital, UK

"It's a serious message, but written in a wonderfully friendly way.

I LOVE the book. I think the questions and spaces for answers is a clever move, as they forced the message to sink in better. Had the layout been any different, my mind would have been conditioned to charge on reading and probably forgetting, but rather it forced me to pause and reflect, making me realise that I need to take better care of my feet."

Mercedes Leal
Author of *The Miracle Code*

"Congratulations on your hard work. What a mission!

I am inspired by the work of Peter Allton and Undefeeted. What an extraordinary mission!"

Dr. Nido Qubein
President of High Point University, North Carolina, USA
Business Consultant, Author, Chairman of Great Harvest Bread Company USA

"I have been following Peter's work and entrepeneurial pursuits and have found his skill, knowledge and dedication to be inspiring."

Darshana Ubl
Entrepreneur, Investor, Advisory

"The world needs more people like Peter Allton. I applaud him for all his hard work and efforts. He is changing the world for the better one healthy foot at a time."

Jason Evers
Entrepreneur, International Speaker, Business Coach, Fort Myers, USA

"Peter and his Undefeeted team are relentless in their pursuit to conquer diabetes and in particular lower limb amputations. I cannot speak more highly of Peter's work ethic and commitment to changing the course of this disease."

Tim Deveson
Podiatrist, Australia

"It is evident when working with Peter that his passion for Undefeeted shines through in everything he does. He is an inspiration to all who know and work with him."

Tina Roberts
UK

"The stats after an ulcer were very sad and we, the people, don't know this, so bringing this out in the book is very important, along with the comparison of breast cancer, prostrate cancer, vrs diabetes is also astonishing, in which Peter brings this to life. Here in the States, we have the AMA (American Medical Association). If you could get feet to be checked as a annual checkup-like eyes, dentist, mammograms, pap smear, what a change that could make?"

Carolyn Thompson
Dental health professional, mother of two, grandmother of six
California, USA

"Peter is a true gent and after reading his book it has opened my eyes and mind to the importance of footcare, especially with diabetes. I have learnt so much from this book, it has also made me realise the consequences and the impact that lack of knowledge can have. Undefeeted is changing that by raising awareness, educating people like you and me, which will in turn prevent suffering and will ultimately save lives. Thank you so much Peter for this amazing book of knowledge, facts and ways to move forward in life in a positive healthy way."

Alison Ford, a happily (now informed and empowered) wife of a type 2 diabetic, UK

"Thank you for being a great inspiration and mentor. I'm so pleased to be able to help educate and raise awareness to empower individuals to stay in the diabetic sweet spot."

Alecia Erdeman
Podiatrist, UK

"As a podiatrist in training, with a passion for public health, I think every podiatrist should join forces with Undefeeted to help make a global change by helping people to be educated about the importance of taking great care of their lower extremities."

Vinit Shah
Temple University School of Podiatric Medicine. Philadelphia, USA

"Peter has taken an event that could have been a family disaster and turned it around to help the wider diabetic community. Well done to him and his lovely wife, Tina, for creating Undefeeted™. Hopefully the awareness you are raising will change the lives of millions."

Debbie Delves
Clinical Director, Dulwich Podiatry Ltd, UK

"I loved the tick boxes: great! Love the make a date in your diary afterwards - very cool. Like the humour – nice context. Like the idea of the companion to online. I think this could be something great!"

Drew Browne
Australia

"As someone whose career of 34 years has been dedicated to treating active foot ulceration and helping to try and prevent amputations in people with diabetes, I applaud Peter for his passion in bringing Undefeeted™ to life. I have witnessed his journey along the way with the long hours and dedication entailed in writing the book "Undefeeted" by Diabetes which is at the core of the Undefeeted™ campaign. The book itself is written in a down-to-earth way that should help any reader by giving them the vital knowledge of how diabetes can affect their feet, or the feet of their loved one.

Furthermore, as the reader progresses they will develop an all important understanding of how specifically they are at risk themselves of foot complications. This awareness and the knowledge found within the book are critical to a person getting into what Peter refers to as the "Diabetic sweet spot".

The book is not a stand alone product and Peter aims to make resources accessible to people of all walks of life and social standing by offering both free and paid for online resources.

Additionally, he is encouraging colleagues around the world to give up a bit of time for people to be able to access free diabetic foot checks which are so critical to helping them truly understand the personal risk they are at.

A final all important third factor to ensure you are truly living safely within the diabetic sweet spot is making sure you act on what you have learnt. Peter says that he didn't take all the effort writing the book just to set up people to fail but that he really wants to transform their lives for the better by keeping them able to do the things they enjoy with those they love. To that end, he has set up support services online to help you get the most from it. In my view, he is spot on when he says that most people including himself need a mentor/ coach to help them change the habits of a lifetime. Indeed he is prepared to walk the talk and has me keeping him accountable on his personal journey with diabetes.

I believe that Undefeeted will truly make a difference to the quality of life of people with diabetes worldwide and so will on a global scale dramatically help to reduce the number of diabetes related lower limb amputations that take place. Here's to slashing the number from the current rate of one every 20 seconds, to one every minute by 2025. That will mean from 4320 per day to 1440 per day.

I wholeheartedly lend my voice to the support of Undefeeted and urge you to do likewise."

Duncan Stang
Diabetic foot coordinator for Scotland

"Undefeeted."TM
by Diabetes

A Step-by-Step guide to keep
your feet healthy for life

Peter Allton
www.undefeeted.org

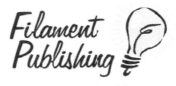

Published by
Filament Publishing Ltd
16, Croydon Road, Waddon, Croydon,
Surrey, CR0 4PA, United Kingdom
Telephone +44 (0)20 8688 2598
Fax +44 (0)20 7183 7186
info@filamentpublishing.com
www.filamentpublishing.com

© Peter Allton 2015

The right of Peter Allton to be identified as the author
of this work has been asserted by him in accordance with the
Designs and Copyright Act 1988.

ISBN - 978-1-910125-10-6

Printed by CPI Antony Rowe

This book is subject to international copyright and may
not be copied in any way without the prior written
permission of the publishers.

Dedication

"To my wonderful daughter Jasmine who I hope and pray will always walk safely within the diabetic sweet spot, and to my family in appreciation of all their support both of my living with diabetes and putting up with me whilst writing this book."

Contents

Part One:
Why People with Diabetes Need to Wake Up!

Part Two:
How to Defuse the Diabetic Time-Bomb.

Part Three:
T.E.A.M – Together Everyone Achieves More.

Quick reference guide.

Foreword:

Dr Gerry Rayman.

Diabetic foot complications are the most costly of all diabetes related complications, and the commonest reason for a person with diabetes to be admitted to hospital. Diabetic foot complications are associated with considerable suffering, and a markedly shortened life span.

Given these concerns and that people with diabetes fear amputation above all other complications, it is astonishing how few people with diabetes know of their personal risk of developing a serious foot complication and what they should do to prevent it. It is policy in the UK for all patients with diabetes to have an annual foot assessment by a trained health care professional. Sadly, only half of patients report that they have had their feet examined, only a third of those are aware of whether they are at high, moderate or low risk of running into a serious foot problem and most do not know what to do if a problem arises. The preventative message is clearly not getting out to health care professionals or to patients.

Peter Allton in this inspiring book turns the table. He puts the person with diabetes in the driving seat. He enthusiastically tutors and encourages the reader to take control by understanding the condition, knowing what care to expect and what to ask for from their health care professionals, and most importantly he kindly reminds them that their responsibility is not only to themselves but also to their loved ones.

This passion is clearly driven by his personal experience of people with diabetes in whom early prevention would have made a difference. Some of this experience is interspersed throughout the book presented as anecdotal cases which promote the reader to reflect on their own condition.

Peter's passion is also driven by personal experience of type 2 diabetes and type 1 diabetes in his young daughter. This book is only one step in his global campaign to raise awareness and empower people with diabetes to prevent this devastating complication. It is a privilege to be invited to write this foreword.

Dr Gerry Rayman

Specialist medical advisor to Diabetes UK and clinical lead for their Diabetes Foot Campaign.

Head of Service

Diabetes Centre, Ipswich Hospital NHS Trust

Foreword:
Fouad I. Ghaly, MD.

When fellow physician and founder of Undefeeted™, Peter Allton, asked me to review a book he was authoring, I wasn't certain what to expect. Yet another book containing diabetes facts? Lists of diabetes buzz words? More patient case studies?

What I found instead was a unique step-by-step guide to creating an action plan that will truly have you living in the "diabetic sweet spot" – the best possible position to manage your diabetes most effectively.

Peter's informative book contains dozens of "aha moments" that will have you thinking, "Why haven't I heard this before?" You will be empowered to take control of your diabetes like never before so that you can continue to live a healthy and active life.

With over 27 years of experience as a Podiatrist, Peter has treated thousands of patients with diabetes. His first-hand patient experience uniquely positions him to identify life-threatening behaviors that are part of many people's everyday life. Finally! A book that conveys the fact that what patients feel, practice, and do in everyday life is critical to successfully controlling this epidemic.

The principal message of this book is that you have the power to directly impact your own vitality and longevity! Each chapter contains exercises to enhance your understanding of the information you'll be learning and to help you develop a personalized road map to live your healthiest life possible.

I am excited about Peter's interactive approach to keeping your feet healthy for life. In addition to the exercises, he has strategically placed tick boxes throughout the margins of this book which make it convenient for you to mark new things you've learned. He also offers convenient online resources and access to life health coaches that will help spur you on to success.

Peter has listened to his patients – and their bodies – for nearly three decades. Isn't this how we doctors truly get to know what works and what doesn't? The information age means patients can quite easily know much more about certain aspects of health management than even their own doctors. Rather than simply dismiss what they have discovered, Peter teaches us to embrace these experiences and learn from them so our patients can live in the diabetic sweet spot.

Fouad I. Ghaly, MD
Regenerative Medicine Physician

Part One:

Why people with diabetes need to WAKE UP!

(Do you know just how much you stand to lose?)

In an average life, our feet walk us five times around the world and yet most of us take them for granted.

People with diabetes simply cannot afford such a lax attitude: **every 20 seconds somewhere in the world a person with diabetes is undergoing an amputation. In many cases, this surgery could have been prevented.**

I wrote *Undefeeted* because I want people to wake up and take control of their condition so that they can continue to live active, healthy, fun lives for many years to come.

And it all starts with the Sweet Spot...

Chapter 1:
The diabetic sweet spot.

The purpose of *Undefeeted* is to help people with diabetes (or their carers/ parents/ family) to understand and accept the risks that the condition poses to their lower limbs. It aims to give you an action plan which will enable you to live in what I call the **diabetic sweet spot**.

Those who should most benefit are people who have already been diagnosed with the disease or know that they are at risk of developing it. Additionally it is a valuable resource for anyone caring for an elderly relative or parenting a child with diabetes.

Providing they put into practice the principles within, the person with diabetes will be empowered to change their lifestyle, take control of their condition and thus positively influence their destiny. You have the power to directly impact how long you will be able to remain active doing the things you enjoy with those you love and ultimately how long you are likely to live.

The sweet spot.

By diabetic sweet spot I mean that you will have put yourself in the best possible place to live safely with your diabetes. My life with diabetes has helped me realise that there are three factors we need to take seriously in order to live with the least risk of developing complications. These factors can be applied to every aspect of diabetes be it diet, exercise, taking your medication, or foot care.

The sweet spot values:

1. Knowledge about your condition.
2. Awareness and acceptance of your personal risk.
3. Taking appropriate action.

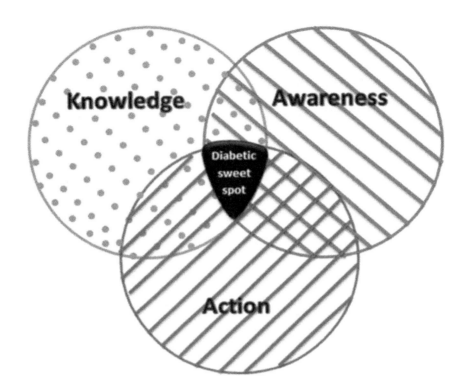

The Diabetic Sweet Spot

So you could for example apply it to *knowing* what to eat, *accepting* the risk to your blood sugars if you eat certain things and then *taking action* to ensure you don't eat them. Likewise it may be the *knowledge* that thickened toenails could ulcerate and lead to infection and then becoming *aware* that you are at risk because you have a thickened nail.

Knowledge and awareness don't keep you safe by themselves. You have to add the magic ingredient – taking action. So in our second example, you could get your nails thinned down by a professional. Once you've taken that step, then and only then are you in the sweet spot for that particular issue.

The diabetic sweet spot is a process rather than a place – you can stay there in safety by choosing to do the right things or you can leave at any time. That depends on your choices and your way of life. Always make sure you stay safe by learning, applying what you learn to your situation and then acting.

It is important to understand how complex foot structure is, how they function and just what they are expected to do every day. Our feet bear the weight of every step of our life's journey. Whether we live with diabetes or not they are vital to our health and wellbeing, but too frequently they are neglected. This neglect often leads to arthritic changes and deformities, amongst numerous other problems. Although debilitating for a non-diabetic, these common issues can become limb and even life-threatening in a person with diabetes.

> *Undefeeted* aims to help you understand the risk you are at now and what can go wrong in the future. It will also help you plan how best to live for the future. By the end of the book you should have started to change your mindset and therefore your lifestyle – ensuring you minimise any chances of developing problems in the future.

How to work with this book.

This is not a book to read and then forget: I want you to use it to transform your life with diabetes for the better. Critical to this is you getting into and remaining in the sweet spot. So I've added exercises in each chapter to help you retain the information you'll be learning – and to help map your personal route to the safety zone of the sweet spot.

You will see tick boxes in the margins throughout this book. Have a pen with you as you read and use the tick boxes to mark the new things you've learned, what you've become aware of about your feet, and the things you've decided to start (or stop) doing. Please do this as you read along.

At the end of each chapter you will find a short exercise where you'll be asked to note the one most important fact you've learned, the main risk factor you've become aware of and the first thing you intend to do or stop doing. All you'll need to do is take a look at the boxes you've ticked throughout the chapter and use them to complete the exercise. (If you're reading the eBook please make sure to get a notebook or set up a document on your PC. It's important that you work through the exercises too).

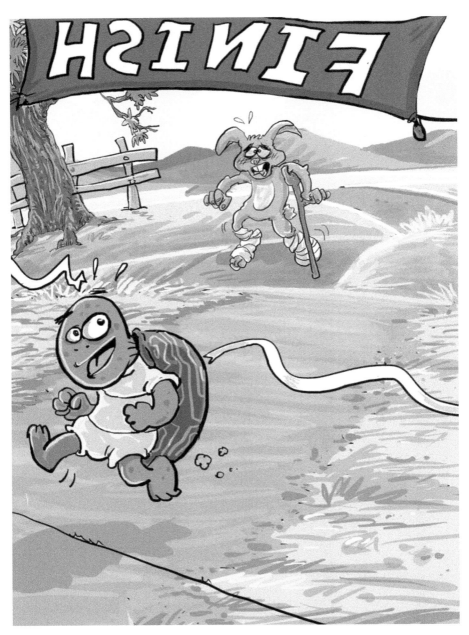

You're on a journey. Pace yourself!

I'd be surprised if you only ticked three boxes in each chapter – you'll probably have far more than that. But rather than overwhelming yourself, let's keep it simple and take it one step at a time. It's better to get one thing right before moving on to the next. Don't be like the hare rushing off to do it all, only to burn out and lose your commitment. Remember that the tortoise always passes the winning line first.

When you've finished the book set a date in your diary for the following month. When the time comes go back to those tick boxes and choose another three to work on for each chapter. You can do this by yourself but it would be far more effective if you worked with a friend or family member. They would become your 'accountability buddy' which I'll tell you more about later.

Sweet spot groups
A whole group of accountability buddies would be even better. My personal experience and that of my patients has taught me that there is power in numbers. Just think of the help and support you'd get if you regularly met up with other people with diabetes who were also working their way towards the sweet spot. And you would be able to help them too.

I hope that in time there will be sweet spot groups dotted around in local communities. They will be a safe place for people to share their difficulties, inspire others with their successes, offer support during hard times and generally help one another along the sometimes difficult road of living successfully and safely with diabetes. As you read on you will increasingly see the benefit and need for this.

Until such time as my vision becomes a reality, you can find all the support you need online at **www.undefeeted.org/forum**.

As you progress through this book you can expect to:
1. Gain in-depth knowledge which will enable you to intervene and reduce the risk of complications developing.
2. Understand what action to take should a complication develop.
3. Learn to accept that because you have diabetes you are at a heightened risk of limb-threatening complications.

4. By carrying out some of the suggested activities, you'll become aware of any specific complications that are already posing a threat to you.

5. Learn that knowledge, acceptance and taking the right action will put you in the safest possible position – the sweet spot. By choosing to do whatever it takes to live in the sweet spot, you have the absolute best chance of living a long healthy life doing the activities you enjoy with those you love. Follow the advice in *Undefeeted* and diabetes won't have a chance to devastate your quality of life.

This book doesn't stand alone; it's a companion to the online campaign of the same name (**www.undefeeted.org**). Here you'll find many resources and a coaching programme so that you can truly get the most out of the book's content. Use the two together and give yourself a fighting chance to remain in the sweet spot.

Undefeeted aims to see more people in control of their diabetes able to live active healthy fun lives for many years to come with the result that globally the number of diabetes-related amputations will reduce dramatically, putting the current shocking statistics firmly in the past.

Chapter 2:
Are your feet killing you?

Life is a rollercoaster: we've all had experiences that brought us pleasure and happiness and others that have plunged us into despair and misery. One of those big dips could have been finding out that you or someone you love has diabetes.

If its type 2 then it's often a gradual process: we trundle along and discover that we're pre diabetic (or as it was called previously, borderline). We may not take the threat seriously. That's one of the huge dangers of type 2 diabetes because you can live with it for many years without being aware you have it and yet all the time the elevated blood glucose will likely be affecting your body, particularly your feet, eyes, kidneys and cardiovascular system. Maybe you were diagnosed from a routine blood test having presented with some of the common symptoms of thirst, tiredness and going to the loo more frequently.

Some diagnoses are more shocking than others and this is usually the case with type 1. Take for example my 11-year-old daughter. Just three days before starting secondary school on a routine visit to the doctor she was diagnosed and put on insulin. It was her diagnosis rather than my own that shook me up so much that it prompted me to create the global Undefeeted™ campaign and write this book.

I live with diabetes and as part of my job as a podiatrist I've seen firsthand the devastating effects it has on the feet and lower limbs. I'll always recall one day when as a relatively newly qualified practitioner I was working in a hospital's diabetic foot clinic. This day left a mark on me because it was the first time I encountered gangrene – in quite a spectacular way...

My first patient was waiting when I returned from a rushed lunch. I'd already been alerted that this was an interesting case involving gangrene so as I walked past I made a point of studying him. He was wearing a smart suit and a gleaming oxford brogue on his right foot. His left foot however was encased in a bedroom slipper that looked about four sizes too big. As an extra touch the front of the upper had been cut away.

I settled him on the patients' couch and began to cleanse his foot making sure I didn't disturb the big toe on his left foot, which was dry and black. It reminded me of the Egyptian mummies in the British Museum. My patient didn't seem too bothered by it. I learned that he'd been coming to the clinic twice a week for several months and was far more upset about the amount of time he had to take off work.

As I gently dressed the diseased toe I realised that it was loose and the next thing I knew I was holding half of it in my hand! The gangrene had effectively auto amputated it. I don't know if it was this that shocked me most or the fact that it could happen to someone in the prime of their working life. Either way that experience made an indelible imprint on my life and career.

So I think you'll understand why I so desperately want to raise your awareness and educate as many people as possible worldwide on the threat diabetes presents to your lower limbs .There's a saying I hear regularly: 'my feet are killing me'. For a diabetic, that saying could be the literal truth. ❏

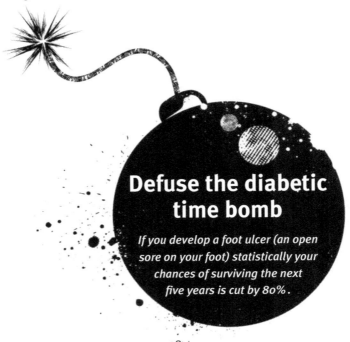

Defuse the diabetic time bomb

If you develop a foot ulcer (an open sore on your foot) statistically your chances of surviving the next five years is cut by 80%.

The above is not a widely known fact but just compare it to other conditions which have more fatal reputations.

There are three people in a room: one has breast cancer, one has prostate cancer, and the final one is a person with diabetes who currently has a foot ulcer. What are their chances of not surviving the next five years? The lady with breast cancer has an 18% chance; the man with prostate cancer has a 40% chance. The diabetic with the foot ulcer? They have a shocking 80% chance that they will not survive five years. Yet if these people shared their problem with you, who would you give the most sympathy to?

Hearing that someone has a foot ulcer and has diabetes is likely to go in one ear and out the other for most people. It is time the condition was treated with as much respect as cancer; with resources, research and publicity.

There are three coexisting problems that need to be addressed. If any one of them is ignored the consequences can disrupt your life – even to the point of causing your premature death.

These three problems are:

1. Not having the **knowledge** required to minimise your risk of complications or to deal with pre existing complications.
2. Not **accepting** the risk you are at as someone with diabetes and specifically your personal risk factors.
3. Not taking the right **action**.

Conversely if you tackle these three problems then you will remain in the diabetic sweet spot. I hope this book will help you do that.

Over the past 29 years, I have had almost daily encounters with clients with some level of diabetes-related complications and often they were totally unaware of these problems. Then, four years ago I was diagnosed with it and suddenly diabetes became personal.

My own journey with the illness has helped me realise that you need three key elements if you want to maximise your chance of living successfully with the disease.

1. It's vital that you **know all about your disease**. What are the symptoms, dangers, things to do and things to avoid? ❏
2. You have to **fully accept that you have diabetes** not just on a superficial level but really taking it on board. You are not superhuman; you are at risk and you have to do something about ❏ it. Diabetes is a horrible disease largely because its effects are so gradual that they often go unnoticed – until it's too late.
3. It's no good having the knowledge and accepting you are at risk if you don't **take action** and move yourself into the sweet spot. Getting into and staying in the diabetic sweet spot is critical for ❏ the wellbeing of your feet as well as your future health.

Diabetic foot complications are a clear and present danger and, once wounded, many feet will develop a superficial infection which can rapidly spread to deeper tissues, including the bones, and then go on to require a partial or full foot or lower limb amputation. Your feet can literally be killing you as 80% of diabetes-related amputees don't survive the next five years.

The diabetic sweet spot (see the preceding chapter for a full explanation of this concept) can be applied to all areas of diabetes management. For example, a person with diabetes needs to know what they can safely eat, they need to accept the risks associated with poor glucose control and they need to act by buying the right food and eating the ❏ right amount of it. This of course needs to be balanced with exercise and correct medication if appropriate.

I apply the diabetic sweet spot to all aspects of the condition although this book will primarily focus on foot issues.

Before I expand on the diabetic sweet spot in detail over the next few chapters I want to look at an unconscious assumption that many people seem to have. I call it the 'foot myth'.

The foot myth – feet just aren't that important.

(Please circle YES or NO.)

1. Do you go to the dentist?	**Yes** or **No**
2. If you have children, do you make sure they go to the dentist?	**Yes** or **No**
3. Do you ever get your eyes checked by an optician?	**Yes** or **No**
4. Have you ever had your feet checked?	**Yes** or **No**
5. Are your feet any less important than your teeth or eyes?	**Yes** or **No**

Most of us take it for granted that we will be able to continue doing the things we have always done. People don't realise just what their feet are expected to do or what they will need to be able to do in the future.

Take a moment to think of a time when you didn't have something you took for granted. Perhaps the car broke down, the buses were on strike, or maybe there was a power cut just as you were about to cook the kids' dinner. Have you ever had a broken leg or arm? Was it frustrating (as well as painful)? I bet you suddenly realised how important these things are to you.

If you had prior warning you would do your utmost to take avoiding action, wouldn't you?

The truth is that we can't plan our future: illnesses, accidents, and the gradual process of wear and tear. As we get older we all know we deteriorate physically but even so we don't expect problems later on if all is well at the moment. We think minor nuisance problems are as bad as it gets. I often hear people saying "I'm not that bad yet." Or "it's probably nothing" and the classic "I thought it would go away by itself."

I have people coming to see me who have put up with their 'little niggle' for months and often years. They never thought of doing anything about it. By the time they do decide to visit me their 'niggle' has become a serious problem. This is never more true than in someone with diabetes where delay in getting a problem seen to can have life-changing consequences even leading to amputation.

I don't blame you for not having looked after your feet up to now because no one has bothered to warn you. However from today forwards you have to take on board the seriousness of good foot health especially as you are living with diabetes. You cannot afford to continue being complacent. Your feet need to move up to number one on your priority list, ahead of eyes and teeth.

Why is it that from childhood we're taught to look after our teeth and get our eyes checked and yet our poor feet are overlooked? Think about it: if you don't take your child to have their feet checked no one bats an eyelid, yet if you miss a dental check-up you would be thought of as negligent.

Imagine a child with a lifetime ahead of them, their feet will walk an average of five times around the world and yet they're expected to begin that journey without any check-ups! I often tell parents that their child's verruca is actually a blessing in disguise as it allows me to check for structural issues that could lead to problems for their son or daughter in later life.

I urge you today to make a commitment to yourself to take your feet and those of your loved ones seriously. Don't wait until you experience a problem, be proactive and try to prevent future complications by looking after your feet now and paying them the attention they deserve.

That way you won't succumb to the myth that most people are captive to – that their feet simply aren't important. The foot myth is a lie at every level and especially so for someone with diabetes.

1. What would you most miss if your feet started to develop problems?

....

....

....

....

....

2. If you weren't able to get around without pain, would that have an impact on your job? Your family? Your social life? Your hobbies and interests?

....

....

....

....

....

What about if you weren't able to get around at all? Would that affect your quality of life? How?

....

....

....

....

3. How would you and your family cope if you had to stop work?

....

....

....

....

....

4. How would you cope if you had to have an amputation?

....

....

....

....

....

5. How would your loved ones deal with your premature (and avoidable) death?

....

....

....

....

....

6. Do you think it could be a good idea to start treating your feet as well as you treat your teeth?

YES?   **NO?**

As you will see in the following chapters the feet are one of the most important parts of the body. Frequently, even for someone without diabetes, their feet will either deteriorate themselves or cause ❏ deterioration elsewhere in the body.

This deterioration can become all the more critical when someone develops diabetes. That said it stands to reason that as all of us hope to live a long active life and none of us know for sure if we are destined to develop the condition, we should place a lot more importance on looking after our feet. This will help us continue to lead a normal active life whether or not diabetes is a part of our future.

Exercise: get into the sweet spot

What I want you to do right now is revisit the tick boxes in this chapter and answer the questions or complete the statements below.

1. What is the most important thing that you have learned in this chapter?

....

....

....

....

2. Which main risk factor have you become aware of?

....

....

....

....

3. The one big thing I am going to start/stop doing is

....

....

....

....

If you need to break that down into several steps, please go ahead and note them below. Make sure to add the date by which you intend to achieve each of those steps.

....

....

....

....

Chapter 3:
Knowledge is power.

Knowledge is vital to our existence and survival. We are born more helpless than animals, many of them having the ability to stand shortly after birth. As any parent will tell you, it's a relief when a child learns to walk and talk, to sit up and generally become more independent. But a parent or older person has to teach the child what to do.

As a person who is starting a new life with diabetes, it is vital that you have a positive attitude towards learning as well as having someone to teach you about the condition and what you can do to help yourself. It's best if you look to an expert for your information. With ❏ babies and children, parenting books, grandparents, and friends with children can be invaluable. It's just the same with diabetes – it is best to learn about your condition and its associated risks from an expert and people with experience. It would be silly taking time to listen to someone (including yourself) if they don't know much about diabetes. In the course of this book I will introduce the idea of diabetic sweet spot groups which will give you a perfect opportunity to gain as well as share a wealth of knowledge. Or you could go to ❏ **www.undefeeted.org/sweetspot** for more information if you'd like to find out right now.

It's a pretty safe bet that you paid very little attention to your feet until you picked up this book or until you developed diabetes. In the 6,000-plus people of all ages surveyed by Circle Podiatry more than 80% had never visited a podiatrist or had any professional input on how to look after their feet. *Undefeeted* aims to give you comprehensive knowledge about feet and what can go wrong with them. More importantly, it will help you understand your own feet and how diabetes can affect them – or may already be affecting them.

As a podiatrist I am aware of the dangers and complications of diabetes. Yet four years ago my blood sugars tipped over from having borderline diabetes to becoming type 2 diabetic. This was after approximately 10 years of having annual glucose tolerance tests. Becoming diabetic has made me acutely aware of the need for early intervention in addressing a poor foot structure thereby minimising the devastating effects the disease can have on your life.

I am also extremely aware of the denial aspect so I am not preaching a holier than thou message. I struggle with eating the right things, I find myself working hard and getting into a vicious cycle of working late, getting home just in time to have dinner with the family and put the kids to bed, going to bed late, getting up early, going to work ❏ and always intending to exercise daily... but not always managing it. Additionally it is not uncommon for a person to live with diabetes for several years before being diagnosed. In fact the International Diabetes Federation estimates that 50% of people living with diabetes are unaware they have the disease. If you were living with diabetes but unaware of it for some time before actual diagnosis then it is likely that your elevated blood sugars could already have done damage to your blood vessels and nerves.

> **The International Diabetes Federation estimates that 50% of people with diabetes are unaware they have the disease.**

Even if you were diagnosed very soon after developing the condition or if you are only borderline at present, you may already have walked the equivalent of three times around the world and, just like a well-used car, your feet (and probably other parts of the body such as your knees, hips and back) will already be showing some deterioration ❏ even if you are not fully aware of it.

❏

Look down at your feet right now. Take your shoes and socks off and look at them (if you're reading this on the train wait till you get home, but do it this evening while it's still a fresh idea in your mind – in fact go ahead and set an alarm on your phone or write it down somewhere to remind you).

Now that you're looking at them would you say they are gleaming Ferrari or over-the-hill bangers? If you're over the age of 10 the chances are that there will already be some deterioration and the older you are the more attention you will need to give them not just to keep them going but also to prevent more serious problems later on in life.

If you have diabetes then multiply the importance of that last statement by 100 and you'll be getting close to just how crucial it is that you look after your own feet.

Here in the UK it is a legal requirement to have an MOT[1] test if a car is more than three years old. If I still had the first car I ever owned by now it would have had about 20 MOTs and 40 services along with countless spare parts.

Why do we think our bodies are immune to the passage of time? We see our parents and grandparents getting older and not being able to do what they once could. We seem to just accept the inevitable deterioration that comes with advancing years without realising that we can do something to help reduce (although not eliminate) the effects of ageing.

Case Study

Bob, an elderly gentleman, was brought to my clinic by his daughter Sara because his nails needed cutting. It was his first visit so I paid attention as he hobbled in on his stick with Sara holding his other arm.

When they got into my room, she gasped when she saw how long his nails were. I could tell that Sara was feeling guilty. But how could she have known what was going on? The only thing she'd ever done for her dad's feet was buy the usual pair of socks for Father's Day and the slippers he lived in at home. I often come across situations like this where even spouses are unaware of their loved one's foot health.

---

[1]MOT stands for Ministry of Transport.

As I looked closer I saw hard crusts of callus had built up where Bob's joints had become prominent under the balls of the feet. I explained that this had happened as a result of the toes retracting causing claw toes and displacing the natural fatty padding that should normally protect them.

It was at this point that the penny dropped. Sara realised that even though she was 23 years younger than her dad her toes were doing a similar thing.

"Is that why I'm getting a burning feeling?" She asked.

I explained how we often don't have an ideal structure and that it deteriorates over time. I talked about why Bob's big toe joint had developed a bunion and she remarked that she thought hers had come because she used to wear high heels all the time.

"I've never worn high heels!" Bob was a big chap, more than six feet tall and at least 20 stone. He would have been quite a sight in stilettos!

"So I can blame my dad for my feet?"

"We certainly inherit our foot structure although often it can skip generations and be a mixture of both parents. Then there are external factors such as pressure whilst in the womb, accidents in early life and of course wearing unsuitable shoes. So wearing high heels may well have exacerbated your bunions and made them appear earlier than they would otherwise."

"I used to love wearing them. I never imagined I was going to end up like dad. Do you think they'll get as bad as his – is it inevitable?"

"The earlier you get sensible about what you are wearing and address the foot structure the better. You can't reverse the deterioration, but hopefully you can slow it down. We can help by providing special insoles called orthotics and you can help yourself by wearing them and choosing more sensible shoes for everyday life. Then when you have a special occasion you should be comfortable in your heels."

"My daughters are 17 and 12; how do I help them? The 17-year-old loves heels and I can already see some redness over the same joint."

"It's always difficult with kids, especially girls, but maybe you could let them see your feet? You could complain a bit; that could be a way to bring up the topic without them feeling that you're lecturing them."

"If I showed them my feet that'd scare the life out of them," Bob winked at Sara.

"My kids often see photos in my text books that I accidentally on purpose leave out at home... It does more for raising their awareness than any lecturing I can do."

Sara nodded.

"Then I suggest bringing them in to see a podiatrist as early as possible even if there aren't any problems yet. It makes them aware of the importance of looking after their feet. You'll be doing them a huge favour," I said.

The rest of Part One goes into why it's so important to be aware of your risk on a more personal level and then the importance of taking action in order to stay in the diabetic sweet spot.

Parts Two and Three will give you the knowledge you need to fight the effects of the disease. You cannot be in the sweet spot without all three components so please continue gaining knowledge by reading on, try to relate it to yourself personally by understanding the risk you are at, and then commit to taking the necessary action. So make sure to tick the boxes when you come across something that is relevant to you and please commit to doing the exercises at the end of each chapter.

Why the diabetic foot is like a fort.

We have some amazing castles in the UK that were built centuries ago. A key point in their design was to make them strong so they would protect the people living within. Some castles may never have been assaulted and others may have remained peaceful for many years before an enemy attacked.

Later in the book you will discover how similar your feet are to a fort or castle: how they are designed to defeat enemy attacks. Just as a castle would have been safe from attack during peaceful years, so too you may have lived your life to date with no apparent problems – but that doesn't mean you won't experience an attack one day... In ❏ Part Two I'll explain what form those attacks may take, what defence mechanisms you need, what defence mechanisms may be out of order and how to protect against an attack if it comes.

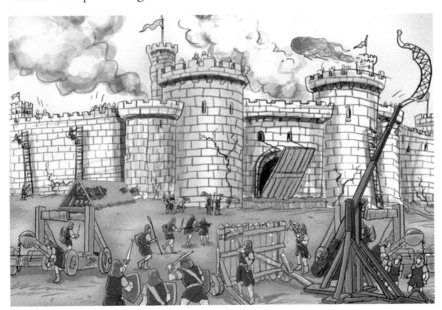

How are the defences of your ~~fort~~ feet?

You are going to learn how to be the captain or commander of your feet and how you are responsible for their downfall or success in any of the battles that may come. Crucially you will also learn how to pre- ❏ empt and avoid many of the attacks.

Just as a castle needs maintenance to remain strong so too you should look after your feet throughout life rather than just fighting off attacks when they occur. Keeping your feet in good condition will help negate the effects of any assault on them in the future. ❏

A castle's foundations need to be strong. So too your foot structure needs to be strong, able to support the whole body and to withstand whatever is thrown at it. ❏

The castle walls are like your skin and need to be able to endure any attacks from the enemy. Any break in the walls leads to a greater risk of invasion (i.e. infection). These attacks can be in the form of one big ❏
event or injury or they may be less severe but more repetitive, which means that the wall (skin) finally gives in to the continual pressure.

The lookouts within need to be aware of any attack so they can raise the alarm. If they were killed, new soldiers would take their place. Likewise if your sensitivity to pain is affected you need to put in place ❏
a means of being aware of any danger.

Most importantly of all the castle needs a leader to strategise its defence – you need to step up and be that leader becoming aware of ❏
any potential attacks and any weaknesses in your defence that may predispose you to attack.

How to get the most out of this book.

It's estimated that when you read something for the first time you only retain a pathetic 10-20% of the information. I didn't put all this effort into writing so you'd only get that small proportion of the facts into your head! Here are some proven ways to help you to retain the knowledge you learn – you would do well to implement them for any important reading matter.

The following techniques will help you retain more than 10-20% of the information in this book:

- Writing down your learnings will help. ❏
- Or draw pictures to illustrate what you have read. ❏

- Tick the boxes that are relevant to you as you go along. Tick the things you've learned, the risks you feel apply to you, and the actions you should take. ❏
- Teaching someone else what you have learned not only helps them but consolidates the information for you. You could talk to someone else with diabetes or maybe a family member who, by learning about it, will be able to help you. ❏
- Doing the same in groups can be a really valuable way to get things to stick in your mind. ❏
- Put the things that you have learned into practice. ❏

By the time you have finished reading this book you should have all the knowledge you need to live safely in the diabetic sweet spot. But knowledge alone won't prevent diabetic foot complications or even ❏ an amputation.

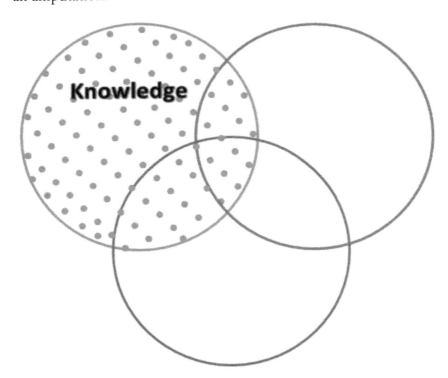

As you progress through the book, I encourage you to participate in the interactive exercises and to write down your learnings so you will

have a much better chance of remembering them. Just writing things ❏
down helps us to remember, but actually doing the things you learn
will help you retain it forever.

That said your circumstances may differ in a year or two's time and
Undefeeted should be kept as a resource you can dip into in later years
to top up your knowledge or get advice in an emergency. The more
effort you put into retaining the information the more you will be
able to help yourself and others.

Later in the book I encourage you to find a buddy who will have a
good understanding of your situation. This again helps you retain the
knowledge better. Likewise I would encourage you to set up or join
a sweet spot group where you get to learn from each other, anything
from new recipes to what has helped you with diabetic neuropathy. ❏
We will be compiling a list of sweet spot groups so please visit
www.undefeeted.org/sweetspotgroups for more information.
Alternatively you could join the diabetic sweet spot forum and
in time form a more personal group from there. Please visit ❏
www.undefeeted.org/forum.

Exercise: get into the sweet spot.

What I want you to do right now is revisit the tick boxes in this
chapter and answer the questions or complete the statements below.

1. What is the most important thing that you have learned in this
   chapter?

....

....

....

....

....

2. Which main risk factor have you become aware of?

....

....

....

....

....

3. The one big thing I am going to start/stop doing is

....

....

....

....

....

If you need to break that down into several steps, please go ahead and note them below. Make sure to add the date by which you intend to achieve each of those steps.

....

....

....

....

....

Chapter 4:
Change your mindset, change your life.

To truly get into the sweet spot you will probably need to shift your mindset. In my experience of treating patients with diabetes the biggest single problem (second only to lack of good blood glucose control) is that they often can't grasp the disease's potential to wreak massive damage, especially in their lower limbs but also in their ❑ bodies generally.

Mindset is important on two levels:

1. You have to grasp how important your feet are.
2. You must understand that as a person with diabetes your feet are ❑ at risk. That risk could be imminent danger to your feet or a long-term risk of problems developing later in life. ❑

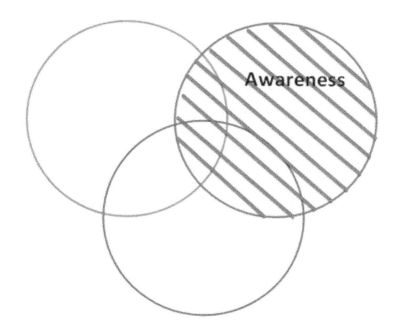

I recently had the pleasure of speaking with a blind person who does incredibly well at getting around. We were at a party and I realised that a rug we were standing on had a big crease in it that could easily trip him if he stepped back. I pointed it out and the evening ended without mishap. That situation has a lot of parallels to someone who is in effect blind to the risks diabetes brings them. Firstly he was not aware of the imminent risk even though he knew that he was always more at risk of a trip than someone who could see such hazards. Likewise as a person with diabetes you may have a superficial knowledge of the effects of the disease without having learned of any ❑ personal dangers to yourself.

Once told about it the gentleman at the party wisely listened to the advice and made a note not to step back. Likewise you can choose whether to accept the things you learn about your condition and ❑ whether you do anything about it or not.

You may already have developed unhelpful attitudes about your illness and you may find yourself slipping into one of them as you read this book. Be on your guard against any of them as they all increase your risk.

They are:

1. **Fear.** Fear has two meanings: You have a choice to Forget ❑ Everything And Run **or** Face Everything And Rise. It's often fear of the unknown, the person may not know about the disease or they may not know what to do. The fact that you are reading this is great because many of your fears will be dispelled as you learn what you can do to minimise your risk. So at the end of this chapter and throughout the book you will best combat fear by getting up and acting on what you have learned.

"Inaction breeds doubt and fear. Action breeds confidence and courage. If you want to conquer fear, do not sit home and think about it. Go out and get busy."

Dale Carnegie.

2. **Superhero.** It's very easy when all is going well, maybe when you are young or newly diagnosed, to believe that the worst will never happen to you. Not everyone with diabetes will get lower limb complications but there is a massively increased risk and it doesn't go away just because you're okay at the moment. Diabetes, if not controlled, will silently be affecting your body and foot problems are probable. ❑

3. **Blasé.**

> *"There are no wishy-washy astronauts. You don't get up there by being uncaring and blasé. And whatever gave you the sense of tenacity and purpose to get that far in life is absolutely reaffirmed and deepened by the experience itself."*
>
> Chris Hadfield.
> Astronaut
> Former Commander of the International Space Station.

Becoming an astronaut is reserved for but a few, yet we are all on a journey that can take us to amazing places. I am not talking about geographical locations but your life experiences. If you embrace ❑ the sweet spot values, you will find that the life experience they bring you will reaffirm the importance of the decision you made to take your diabetes seriously.

4. **Can't accept it.** The times I have felt this way are most likely to be when I have a sense of 'woe is me'. I have become self-focused rather than seeing that there are others involved – parents, friends ❑ and kids who are likely to be affected by my moping around. Rather it is better to focus on being giving towards others. This is easier said than done but try it and you may just see that gradually you don't feel quite so bad about your own situation.

5. **Apathetic.** Being apathetic about your condition is really being selfish towards those who love you. It is like looking your child or loved one in the eye and saying: "I don't love you enough to ❑ take control of my diabetes and do all I can to have as healthy and long a life as possible."

> *"Apathy can be overcome by enthusiasm, and enthusiasm can only be aroused by two things: first, an ideal, which takes the imagination by storm, and second, a definite intelligible plan for carrying that ideal into practice."*
>
> Arnold J. Toynbee.

I encourage you to think of your ideal future, let your imagination run wild with the things you would like to be able to do in five, 10 or even 20 years' time and then, throughout the course of this book and with support from **www.undefeeted.org**, you will be able to form a sensible solid plan to empower you to attain those goals.

6. **Defeatist** (or should we call it defeetist?) The old saying 'it isn't over till the fat lady sings' comes to mind. In the vast majority of cases there is no reason to be defeatist. You may just need a different perspective or some encouragement to try something else. For some having a buddy or being part of a group where they learn they are not alone can make all the difference. Thomas Edison can teach us a lot about persevering at times when things feel hopeless. He said that he hadn't had 10,000 failures at producing a successful commercial light bulb – he'd just found 10,000 ways not to do it. His mindset was that every failure took him one step closer to getting it right. I love the other comment he made when asked some years later what he'd be doing now if he hadn't got it right. He answered "I would still be in my lab trying." In our walk with diabetes there is no room for defeatism. We can learn how to live best at any particular stage and whatever risk we are at.

7. **Pessimistic.** As you work through the book you should come to understand which areas are most risky for you. Whether you become aware of imminent danger or of potential future problems, you have two choices on how to deal with this awareness: you can either be negative or positive. Choose to be positive; embrace the challenges that may lie ahead and do your best to understand what you need to do to remain as safe as possible. Pessimism can be defeatist and dangerous. Yes, it can be

difficult sometimes to think positive but in my experience there is a positive side to any negative situation and the more you focus on the positive the more it becomes a reality. If you feel negative or hopeless at any point as you read this book, write it down and think of an alternative positive opposite to it. Then focus on that positive which will over time become more and more real to you until it becomes your predominant thought. For example you may have a foot ulcer and have just read that people with diabetic foot ulcers have an 80% likelihood of not surviving for five years. You could be forgiven for getting depressed about that. However realise that it's not so much the ulcer that's the problem, but more that the person with the ulcer doesn't know what to do and hasn't looked after themselves properly. By reading this book you will be empowered to lead a more healthy life, you'll know what the dangers are, how to prevent their onset and how to deal with them if they occur. So grab hold of all the positives and realise that you are actually better equipped than most people.

I want you to gain a real understanding of the risk you are at because without that you are unlikely to act to save yourself. The majority of us don't place much importance on our feet until they bother us and even then we often put up with the discomfort for a while before seeking help. Some people with diabetes may not feel the discomfort and therefore won't realise they need help until things have got a lot worse; even if their feet haven't deteriorated to this point and they can feel the problem, it is still vital that they get it seen to quickly.

Each of us walks the equivalent of five times around the world and most of us set off on this journey with no long term objectives. During our teens we may get a few ideas and these dreams, plus the ones that come later, influence what we put our bodies and feet through. This thought was highlighted to me recently when I saw a new client. He was a livestock farmer and his feet had been asked to do a lot more than mine. Obviously it's not just work that affects our feet; he could have flopped in front of the TV every evening while I could've been out training for marathons. The point is that what we do will dictate how much we use our feet and consequently that may, if there is an underlying problem, cause complications.

On life's journey you never know what is round the next corner or what may run out in front of you at any time. Why am I writing about the meaning of life in a book about diabetes? What gives me the authority to talk to you about your journey? Well, I'm a podiatrist with 27 years' experience and I've treated more than 200,000 feet. In my profession I talk to people who are unable to continue doing what they want to do. In some cases what they always took for granted has now been snatched away from them. That may be Jenny who at the age of 36 could no longer wear high heels, or maybe James who couldn't join the rest of his family hiking in the Peak District, or perhaps Mary who at 82 finds it almost impossible to walk the small distance to the local corner shop.

Where are you on life's journey?

If you're not in a quiet place I want you to stop reading and pick up the book again when you are because I want you to do something that is simple but very powerful.

Okay so you're back with me, please make yourself comfortable. This may sound a bit woolly but bear with me because countless seminar attendees have testified that this exercise is very useful in life in general. I feel it is even more valuable when you are suffering from something like diabetes. Please have a pen ready to do the exercise that follows.

- On page 53 you will see a long line. You'll see the two unavoidable things that happen to every human being one at each end: birth and death. We don't want to focus too much on the end but nevertheless it's there. Now plot where you are on the lifeline.
- Now close your eyes and spend three minutes thinking of all the things your feet have done for you or the amazing places they have taken you so far in your life.
- Now open your eyes and write down the most important things your feet have enabled you to achieve next to the relevant age on your timeline. It's essential for you to appreciate what your feet have done for you.

Happy Birthday!

10

20

30

40

50

60

70

80

and

beyond...

Goodbye ☹

> *"A goal is a dream with a deadline."*
>
> Napoleon Hill.

- I know you know what's coming next and you may have jotted down goals before, but please spend a few minutes on this. Close your eyes again and imagine what you would specifically like your feet to do for you. It may be strolling along the beach with a loved one, walking your dog, climbing a mountain or simply being able to get to the shops. It could even be to get up and walk to the next room. That is fine as long as your goals stretch you and aren't so vague that you can't find a way to achieve them.

- Now plot those dreams on your lifeline roughly at the point you'd like to achieve them. Although *Undefeeted* is all about keeping you fit and well with two feet intact it's more than that – we want to empower you to be successful in your life. We believe that with the use of our online resources and life health coaches (also known as sweet spot coaches) you will be spurred on to achieve above and beyond whatever your current dreams may be.

Your dream may seem small, but think of the lady who just wished she could get down the stairs of her first floor flat and along the road to the shops. There is always someone worse off than you and you owe it to yourself, your family, friends, and to God to always do your best to live to your maximum potential. ❑

A dream will remain just that unless it becomes a goal and that goal needs to have a deadline by which it is achieved otherwise you'll get distracted and it will never become a reality. We need to make ❑ plans for how to achieve our goals and then and only then if we hold ourselves to account will that dream stand a chance of becoming reality.

> *"If you cannot do great things, do small things in a great way."*
>
> Napoleon Hill.

So with a positive mindset of your life ahead and gratitude in your heart for where your feet have taken you it is now important to fully accept the state they are in and make adjustments to your lifestyle to lessen the effects of any deterioration caused by your diabetes or indeed by the passage of time.

Tell yourself regularly: ❏

- I am at risk (know specifically which risks).
- I am positive.
- I act quickly.
- I want to live this life to the full.

When you think about your own mindset, are you more likely to be pessimistic, blasé or something else? Note it down under the awareness question at the end of this chapter. Then in the action section put in anything you can do to overcome that mindset. This could be having a mentor or buddy to hold you accountable or writing a daily to do list and sticking to it. I recently became aware of the not to do list and have found it invaluable. We're good at focusing on our goals and what we need to do yet we pay little attention to the bad habits and other aspects of life that hold us back. The not to do list focuses on identifying bad habits and negative traits and will help you overcome them.

Exercise: get into the sweet spot.

Have a look at the tick boxes in this chapter and answer the questions or complete the statements below.

1. What is the most important thing that you have learned in this chapter?

....

....

....

....

....

....

2. Which main risk factor have you become aware of?

....

....

....

....

....

....

3. The one big thing I am going to start/stop doing is

....

....

....

....

....

....

If you need to break that down into several steps, please go ahead and note them below. Make sure to add the date by which you intend to achieve each of those steps.

....

....

....

....

....

....

Chapter 5:
Time for action.

In-depth knowledge of what can go wrong only gets us part of the way into the sweet spot as we learned in Chapter Three. In Chapter Four we learned that you need the right mindset if you want to move closer to the sweet spot; most importantly you have to accept that you are more at risk than people without diabetes. In this chapter we will discover the importance of acting on what we have learned which will mean we are right at the heart of the sweet spot and therefore in ❏ the safest possible place.

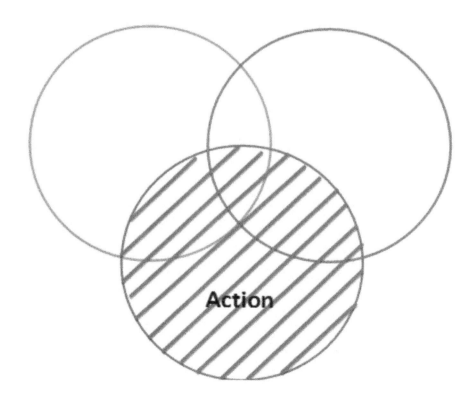

Why not take action?

You would think that once advised of the dangers it would motivate anyone to do what they can to ensure their safety and yet time and again patients return with reoccurrences of problems that would have been less likely to reoccur if only they had acted on the advice they'd been given. The most common is people walking around the house barefoot after being advised not to do so, then coming in with wounds on the bottom of their feet from stepping on something sharp – particularly risky if they have neuropathy as they don't feel it and so don't get it treated quickly, which means infection is likely to set in. Before you know it a 3mm piece of glass has caused an infection that has spread and requires an amputation. How can we let something so small affect us and our family's lives in such a huge way?

Once someone knows about their condition and is aware of the risks that they are at you would think that they would find it easy to act... Take it from me even though I have plenty of knowledge about my specific risk areas and have seen firsthand the horrific sights and suffering of patients with diabetic foot complications, it is still not easy for me to be consistent.

Someone once referred to this lack of action and responsiveness to risk as 'neuropathy of the brain' because it seems as if the person just doesn't feel the danger they are in. Without action all you have learned is useless and not responding to your personal risks is almost making a mockery of your condition and asking for trouble.

What's stopping you?

So why is it that so many people don't take action to achieve their dreams or, in this case, to control their diabetes and safeguard their future? I often find that people haven't taken action because they've never been told that they would benefit from it. Below is a list (it's not exhaustive) that outlines many of the reasons (excuses) people have for not taking action. Add any other ones you can think of and feel free to ❏ contact me via **www.undefeeted.org** so I can include them in further editions of this book.

As you go through use the tick boxes to identify which one(s) apply to you. Then at the end of the chapter you will know what is keeping you out of the sweet spot and you can prioritise an action plan to tackle them. But please be on your guard and resist the temptation to justify or rationalise any of them. If one of the items on the list automatically sends you into justification mode then you can be sure that it is the most important one for you to deal with. Shift your mindset in that area and all the others will follow. One other thing to note is that this whole concept is fluid: it can change over time so your biggest weakness now can become your strength only to be replaced by another weakness later on.

The excuses we use to stop action in its tracks.

1. Too busy.

This really is an excuse and one many of us convince ourselves is real. It makes us feel comfortable that we are doing our best considering the pressure we are under. I've certainly succumbed to it and with a wife, four children, four businesses, two rabbits and commitments to my church, many people would tell me to slow down and not burn myself out. Yet there are always ways to make better use of the time we have. I am making better use of my time now and whatever time management system you put in place you will find you can fit a lot more in. ❏

2. Peer pressure.

I'm not just talking to those of you who are at school. Peer pressure can affect us at any age and can be very subtle. None of us likes to think that we are ruled by others and yet our society and its expectations can literally 'defeat' you. Take for example ladies shoes. Fashion dictates that ladies wear pointed shoes and high heels (let me just say here that this is okay for occasional wear at special events and my wife looks great in them) but don't put up with having to wear them just because you think your boss, colleagues, friends or even your spouse expect it.

Go ahead and think how you may be affected by what others think. Other examples are: eating the wrong food; not exercising;

not wearing slippers (they're not the coolest of attire); and walking ❏ barefoot on the beach.

Peer pressure is a fear of what others are thinking. The acronym of 'false evidence appearing real' should be borne in mind because a lot of the time the other party is not even thinking about you.

I remember my eldest daughter preparing for her school prom. She'd decided that as she loved Converse shoes so much she would make them look extra special and glitzy rather than going along with the crowd (her friends were all wearing high heels). She spent hours preparing them. When the evening came I remember her walking down the stairs and looking so beautiful. I should point out that she was not the one suffering from peer influence, it was me who was conjuring up images of her feeling awkward and out of place.

I dropped her off at school where they were all waiting for the coach to take them to the venue and as I watched all these teenage girls tottering around on ridiculously high heels I consoled myself that at least she wouldn't be likely to end up in accident and emergency with a broken ankle.

Four hours later I waited in my car as the coaches let the children off. I could see my daughter chatting with a group of friends which made me feel better. As she drew nearer I realised she had a crown on her head and a sash over her shoulder – she had been crowned Queen of the Prom. Suffice to say my fears had been proved unfounded and, if you think about them logically, you will find probably most of yours are too.

3. No money.

In extreme cases this may be a factor but often it is an excuse. So what if you can't afford the gym membership? Couldn't you go for a walk or a swim instead? Sometimes we need to think outside the box and prioritise our funds to pay for the membership, the personal trainer, ❏ or for a new pair of running shoes.

4. No knowledge.

For many people is not an excuse but a real reason: they just haven't been taught the importance of it. This book and its accompanying resources both online and through the six-monthly optional coaching programme will mean that you have ample knowledge of what to do to best live with your diabetes. ❑

5. No conviction.

You may not feel the importance of what you have heard so far. I aim to instil in you a conviction that for your sake and your family's sake, you should look after your body and specifically your feet to the best of your ability. ❑

> *"Whatever you do may seem insignificant to you, but it is most important that you do it."*
>
> Mahatma Gandhi.

6. Fear.

One of the best ways to combat fear is to take action, not any old action but specific ones aimed to help you overcome the very thing you fear. Often we don't even know what that is so first of all identify your fears. Consider the following examples:

- Fear of failing.
- Fear of getting a foot ulcer.
- Fear of an amputation.
- Fear of having a second leg amputation.
- Fear of not being able to carry on playing sport.
- Fear of not feeling if you have trodden on something sharp.
- Fear of your kids or loved one being beside your hospital bed.
- Fear of death.

The list could go on. But let's learn to turn that fear into confidence and courage by identifying it, learning what to do to best to avoid it happening and then getting up, going out and getting busy doing the ❑ actions we've identified that need to be done.

7. Despair.

Despair is a horrible place to be and my hope is that within the pages of this book you will find the source of your despair and realise what the antidote is so you can take action and free yourself from that miserable place.

Let me encourage you to try the buddy concept as that will help you if you find yourself failing. Furthermore having a buddy should mean you're forced to take your eyes off yourself and help your friend. It is never a bad thing in times of despair to realise that you can minister to someone else. Acts of service and selflessness have healing properties in and of themselves. ❏

8. Lack of prioritisation.

What's the worst case scenario of how your diabetes could affect you if you don't take the right action? Now give that action its appropriate level of priority. Too often we don't realise what the *real* priorities are because we haven't taken the time to sit down and evaluate. The sweet spot exercise at the end of each chapter and then in Chapter 17 will help you with this, along with your buddy, podiatrist, or coach. ❏

9. Stress.

Stress can lead us to make silly mistakes in the moment and over time it can blur our opinion of what is important. We can spend so long stressing over something that has already happened that it takes our focus off what we should really be doing. Other times we stress about things we can do something about but we haven't got a clue what it is we can do. This is where we take on board the advice from the book: buddies and coaches. ❏

10. Injury.

Injury can be a valid reason for us not being able to take action, but often there are ways around it. For example, you can still swim if you have a foot ulcer so long as you take the right advice and wear the right protective device which will keep your foot dry even while swimming. Don't use an injury as an excuse, speak to your health professional or coach to see what can be done. We are blessed to live in an era when there are so many innovative ideas that can help you. ❏

11. Procrastination.

This is one of my weaknesses and I'm sure my writing coach smiled to herself as she read this! Procrastination can be down to a number of reasons and you will have to identify which best fits you.

It may be the person is not taking it seriously enough; has other things that need to be done more urgently (the problem here is that so-called urgent things will keep coming and seem to be more important than your health).

It may be that you are a perfectionist. This is a big one for me and was highlighted to me while I was writing this book. I've had to accept that I have to let go even though it's not perfect because what use is an unpublished book? It's much better to do my best, get it done and then with feedback from you the reader, I can adapt parts for later editions.

On that note please share any areas on how you feel this book can be improved. You are very welcome to contact me through **www.undefeeted.org**. ❏

12. Lack of accountability.

In business as well as health I find it valuable to have someone keep me accountable. This can be anyone though many people find it is best to have someone emotionally removed, so not a spouse for example. A personal trainer, online coach, buddy or a sweet spot group can hold you accountable. You can even ask your kids or grandchildren to remind you ❏ to wear your slippers or count your carbs. My 6-year-old son recently appointed himself as my accountability buddy and just this evening as I walked through the door after a long hard day, he greeted me with "right daddy get on the treadmill and then I want to see you doing your push-ups." If he hadn't prompted me I wouldn't have got on the treadmill; I'd have said I was too tired. As it turns out, I wasn't.

13. Laziness.

The Bible describes laziness as a sin. Does that mean we can't rest? Of course not, but laziness should certainly not become a way of life. A good benchmark to use is to think to oneself 'what good/should/could I be doing now?' And then do it! ❏

14. Apathy.

Look at the timeline you did earlier and stick a photo of your loved ones next to it – apathy should now be easier to overcome. Also getting into a sweet spot group can help lift your spirits and kill apathy as you work as part of a team. ❏

15. Pride.

> *"A man's pride can be his downfall, and he needs to learn when to turn to others for support and guidance."*
>
> Bear Grylls.

Pride truly does come before a fall and Bear's words are so true in the life of a person with diabetes. However self sufficient you are you need to recognise that you may not know all there is to know about your condition and, even more likely, you probably don't know specifically what your risks are and what you can do about them. Give yourself a bit of praise for being humble enough to pick up this book, but guard your heart as you read through, take the advice given and put it into practice. ❏

Sometimes our pride can get in the way because we feel that what we are being told is insignificant. We need to humble ourselves and realise that we are probably not as expert as the person advising us.

Don't let any excuse defeet you.

Which of the above excuses are holding you back? Make a list now. Let's say you have a list of five weaknesses that are preventing you from taking action. Don't read on until you have put a tick in the tick box for each one. At the end of the chapter you will be revisiting these and choosing the three that are most important to you (one for knowledge, one for awareness of risk and one for action). These will be the ones you will address and conquer in your first month of living in the sweet spot.

The Diabetic Sweet Spot

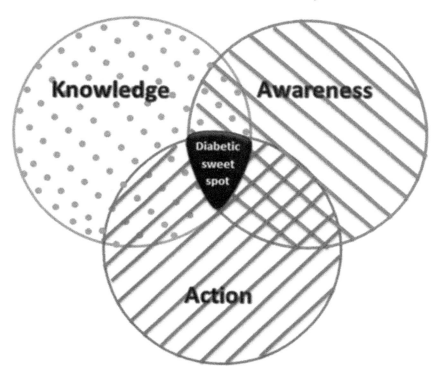

You should now have a clearer idea of what it takes for you to get in the diabetic sweet spot and you may well be feeling a bit overwhelmed by what you have to change. Stick with it, complete the book, and you will find you are empowered to do it all to remain Undefeeted™. Remember, a journey of a thousand miles begins with just one step. The more you get stuck in the further you will go and the easier it will become. So focus on that first step, then the next and the next and so on. Altogether they will allow you to get into – and stay in – the diabetic sweet spot.

> *"That which we persist in doing becomes easier – not that the nature of the tasks has changed, but our ability to do has increased."*
>
> Ralph Waldo Emerson.

We all hope to live long and full lives; we all know that means growing old and that we will experience many wonderful sights on our journey as well as some accidents and illnesses. You may feel you are invincible but the chances are the older you get the more you will feel the need to look after your body as you become aware of the inevitable wear and tear. The feet are not only one of the earliest parts of the body to develop arthritic changes; they can also cause arthritis higher up the body for example in the knees, hips and back. A diabetic with these problems will inevitably become less active and that can lead to higher blood sugar and its associated complications.

A journey of chance

I remember how much planning my parents put into the annual family camping holiday, usually a trip to Yorkshire or Northumberland. The check lists of what to pack, the trailer taking up the garage for about a week before we left as my dad expertly packed it with all the necessities, from the tent to the toilet paper. Then there was the vehicle itself and its service to ensure it was fit for the journey. Tyres were checked and pressures altered to cope with the extra weight.

"Are the connections alright between the car and trailer?"

"Yes dad."

"No, nothing's happening."

So the trailer's brake bulb was checked and changed.

"All working now. Right Peter, help me fill up the windscreen washer fluid."

"Why?"

"So we can see where we're going; if the windscreen gets dirty we can use this to clean it."

Finally in we all piled and off we set. Although we knew where we were heading none of us knew exactly what we would experience in the time that would elapse before we were opening the door of our home again.

"Better just top up the tank," said dad, "that should get us all the way there."

Few of us plan to drive around the world but if we did we'd give it a lot of thought and we'd make sure we had a vehicle fit for purpose. Even just a fortnight trip to Scotland involves quite a bit of planning if you want to make the most of it and those families with more than one car will choose the best one for the job.

The vehicles that transport us most of our life are our feet and we don't have any choice – we are born with what we have and they are expected to cover thousands of miles and carry us for 80 years or so without any problems.

Logic would say that just as you get the car serviced and checked regularly before even a journey of a few hundred miles so too should you get your feet checked, but for the majority of us the answer is 'no, they're not causing me any problems'. Think back to the timeline of your life and work out the number of times around the world you still have to walk. Now realise that when you get up from reading this book those first steps are the start of that long journey. Do yourself a favour: get yourself MOT'd and serviced and look after yourself so you can complete your journey seeing and experiencing everything you want.

I have come to the conclusion that besides lack of awareness the main reason people don't get their feet checked is familiarity. One of my previous neighbours had a great big camper van too big for their drive and each spring it would come out of its winter storage and he'd spend days checking it over in preparation for its summer use. It drove maybe 4,000 miles a year yet it got a tremendous amount of attention. Compare that to my car which I drove on lots of small trips every day: it covered four times as many miles and yet I rarely gave its maintenance a thought.

We don't think of our life as one very big journey, we just get on with it and if something isn't bothering us we don't feel the need to get it checked. Our life is a bit like taking the car out for trips to the local shops day after day. It will wear out and go wrong eventually if we don't look after it; so too with our bodies and in particular our feet.

Life is a journey and a long one at that so don't leave the health of your feet to chance. Every parent should ensure their children's feet are not going to cause problems, as indeed they should do for their own.

Exercise: get into the sweet spot.

It's time to go back over the tick boxes in this chapter and answer the questions or complete the statements below.

1. What is the most important thing that you have learned in this chapter?

....

....

....

....

2. Which main risk factor have you become aware of?

....

....

....

....

3. The one big thing I am going to start/stop doing is

....

....

....

....

If you need to break that down into several steps, please go ahead and note them below. Make sure to add the date by which you intend to achieve each of those steps.

....

....

....

Congratulations on getting to the end of Part One!

Part Two:
How to defuse the diabetic time-bomb

(And what's so special about a diabetic foot anyway?)

The following section aims to give you a comprehensive guide to the complications associated with diabetes and the feet, and the most probable dangers that a person with diabetes could encounter. It will also advise you on how best to keep yourself in the diabetic sweet spot and therefore minimise your risk.

If you already have any of these problems developing you are better off knowing something is wrong so that you can deal with it rather than carrying on under the illusion that all is well – not realising that the fuse to the time-bomb has already been lit. If it has been lit surely it's better to cut the fuse and deal with the problem before it gets worse.

The first chapter will explore the diabetic foot using my fort concept; then we'll break that concept down into the various things that can go wrong with your feet.

Chapter 6:

Why your foot is a fortress.

For centuries kings, queens and leaders would rely on their fortress for protection from enemies. The more hostile a situation the stronger the castle or fort needed to be. Our feet need to be strong too: there is no other part of the body that has to withstand such a hostile environment or such stressful conditions as the foot. ❏

The word fort is derived from the Latin *fortis* meaning strong and the foot is certainly one of the strongest parts of the body. Did you know that it has to withstand one and a half times your body weight being transmitted through it with every single footstep you take? If you run ❏ that increases to more than **three times** your body weight.

Each day the average person walks about 10,000 steps which means that someone weighing 75 kg will put more that 1 million kgs of force ❏ through their feet in one single day. If we take this further, when an average man runs his feet will process more than 112 tons of weight through each limb per mile. It is truly amazing that the foot lasts as long as it does and it's hardly surprising that it usually deteriorates.

Once when I was playing with my son and his toy fort I realised that there are many similarities between forts and feet. I usually get a blank look when I first mention this to patients or colleagues but, once I've explained it, people start to grasp the importance of their feet and – more importantly – what can go wrong, especially if you have diabetes.

We don't give our feet much thought. Even I didn't before being ❏ diagnosed as a diabetic and if I'm truthful it's easy to get caught up in life and, before you know it, you're back in the rut of getting up, sitting on the bed, putting your socks on, shoving your feet into shoes and giving them no more thought until the end of the day when you're in the shower and you give them a quick wash. Out of sight out of mind is the saying that sums up most people's relationship with their feet.

Even when they cause us discomfort and pain we grumble and complain about how our feet are killing us and still we don't do anything about them! I often hear from patients that they have put up with the pain for months or even years before seeking professional help. The general pattern I see is that a person does nothing for a while and puts up with the discomfort, then eventually tries some over-the-counter product before eventually seeking professional help. When a podiatrist sees someone for the first time the client has often put up with unnecessary pain and spent a fair bit of money on ineffective products and, more worrying still, developed a chronic and much harder to resolve problem.

The really scary thing for people with diabetes is that you are at risk of losing the sensation in your feet (this is addressed later in this section in Chapter 10). Pain has been described as a blessing because it warns you that something is going wrong and that you need to take action. Diabetics with neuropathy can no longer rely on pain to give them an early warning.

How your feet are like a fort

First of all they are your foundations. And any building is only going to be as strong as its foundations.

Why did people build forts? In most cases it would have been for protection. The design of the fort was all important: strong, thick, high walls; battlements to protect you whilst allowing you to see out; walkways to get soldiers where they were needed and so on. Imagine there was an assault at the front and all the soldiers were sent to defend it. They don't notice that a second front is attacking from the rear. The enemy targets the door, a natural weak spot, and the attackers notice an area to one side that has not been maintained very well. Again they pour resources into pressurising that area. Finally noticing the attack at the rear, the commander sends some soldiers to defend it, but the walkways weren't built wide enough and are blocked with the debris and bodies from the battle. There's no way through and the rear wall allows the enemy to scale it and overthrow the fort.

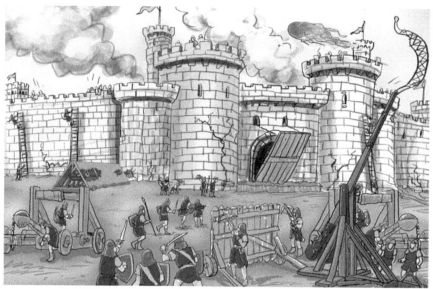

How are the defences of your fort feet?

How the fort was built in the first place will determine its success in keeping its people safe. Similarly we all inherit genes that mean we are born with a particular foot structure and this structure (or specifically problems with it) will determine the types of problems we are likely to encounter later in life. The foot type you inherit can, for example, cause you to end up with bunions, clawing toes or hammer toes.

Your feet will be different to mine and the worse the structure you inherit the more likely you are to develop problems. We will look at how important the foot structure is in the next chapter.

The door of the castle is always a natural weak spot and would be attacked with battering rams. Once the door is damaged by the ram, the enemy can enter and the fort becomes even harder to defend.

Similarly many a foot has been amputated because of a wound forming, for example on the end of the big toe, because the toe is hitting the end of the shoe with every step the person takes. This causes a wound through which the enemy (in our case bacteria) gets in.

A lady came to see me the other day complaining of a sore she had under her big toe. I quickly realised that the problem lay elsewhere in the foot and that this wound was actually being caused by the foot having to compensate for that underlying problem. By addressing the ❏ structural problem we were able to offload the area of high pressure and the wound healed. She was not a diabetic but had she been so the outcome could have been very different.

The attackers of a fort would have looked for weakness in the defences such as cracks in the walls. In the same way infectious bugs will always be loitering and waiting for a weak spot to appear in the form of a ❏ wound or crack in the foot. Then they'll try to invade it.

Once inside the fort the invaders could run riot and overpower the defenders as they struggled to reach the breach in their walls. So too in the diabetic foot. It is as if some of the garrison of defenders are on ❏ leave so when the walls (or skin) are breached the blocked walkways (or blood vessels) don't allow the defensive soldiers (white blood cells) to get to the invading attackers or supplies (nutrients) to reach the defenders in different parts of the fort. In some cases the defenders would be so intent on securing one part of the fort that they wouldn't notice a separate attack in a different area. ❏

A wise captain would appoint watchmen to look out for new fronts in an attack and if the watchmen were killed the captain would immediately send replacements. In the diabetic foot neuropathy may mean that your 'watchmen' are unaware of an attack and the danger it poses. You are the ❏ captain of your fort (I mean foot) and if your watchmen (sensory nerves) are dead then it is your responsibility to become the lookout (i.e. check ❏ your feet daily to ensure there are no signs of attack).

> **"Sincere ignorance is excusable, conscientious stupidity is unforgivable."**
>
> **Martin Luther King.**

Can you see how important your feet are? And yet people take them for granted for years. The big problem is that this level of apathy is engrained in us and as a habit it's not easy to break. ❏

The good news is that you are now aware of the importance of looking after your feet and so have no excuse for continuing to ignore them. You just don't know what you'll hit in the journey of life. People with type 2 diabetes, for example, spent most of their life without the condition and foot health wasn't really on their radar. So although this book is aimed at people with the condition, non-diabetics will be doing themselves a favour by reading on – as the old saying goes, prevention is better than cure. By looking after their feet earlier in life a person sets themselves up to withstand the difficulties their feet will encounter later on, including the challenge of living with diabetes.

Ask yourself the following questions:

(Please circle YES or NO.)

Do I know for sure that my foot structure is alright?	**Yes** or **No**
Could it cause me problems later in life?	**Yes** or **No**
Could that bad back or knee pain have something to do with the way my feet are working?	**Yes** or **No**
What about my kids? Are their feet okay?	**Yes** or **No**

I'll raise your awareness of the issues you face, but thereafter the onus to act is on you! Read, learn and take positive steps so that you can continue living a normal active life doing the things you enjoy with those you love.

To help you take those positive steps, you may find it helpful to join a local diabetic sweet spot group or get an accountability buddy. From time to time you may find vouchers available at **www.undefeeted.org/offers** which will entitle you to a free check-up at an Undefeeted™ preferred podiatry practice.

Your feet and their journey through life.

Your journey through life can be likened to a car journey. The car is supported by four wheels and each one affects its progress. Likewise there are four main factors that affect our feet as we continue our ❏ journey. The diagram will help clarify what I mean.

The four wheels are:

- **Age.** Can't do anything about that, it happens. ❏
- **Activity.** You can choose what you do but the bottom line is we ❏ need to use our feet every day.
- **Footwear.** We can usually choose what shoes we wear although certain jobs may require special kinds of footwear. ❏
- **Foot structure (and its resultant function).** The easiest one to address. We can't change what structure we are born with but we can improve the way it functions and slow down the wear and ❏ tear on our feet.

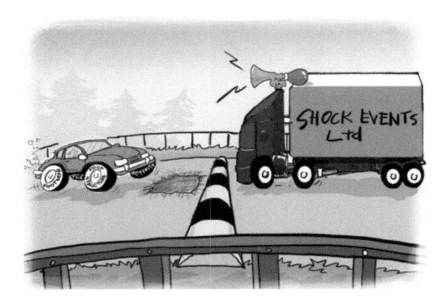

Help make sure your life's journey is as safe as possible

Furthermore, as you continue on your journey from time to time you may hit a bit of a pothole, maybe a twisted ankle or some hip pain or an ingrowing nail. You may hit some speed bumps like forming ❏ bunions or hammer toes which gradually slow you down. Then there ❏ are the major life events which, like a huge articulated lorry bearing down on us in the dead of night, hit us with no warning. These lorries can take the form of life experiences that shake us up maybe leaving ❏ you depressed and not as active as you were, or acute illnesses like a stroke or heart attack, accidents that leave us less able than before or, as we are exploring here, becoming diabetic. ❏

In the following chapters we'll expand on how diabetes affects the feet, but let's just get reacquainted with the concept of the diabetic sweet spot from Chapter One.

As you read on you need to consider whether you are in the sweet spot or not for each of the risk factors that you personally have to deal with. If you ❏ are then think about how you can ensure you stay there. If you are not then work out and **write down** (using the tick boxes and the exercises at the end of each chapter) what it will take for you to find your way there. ❏

To get the most from this book I suggest you read Part Two a chapter at a time, visit the relevant page at **www.undefeeted.org** and watch ❏ the self-help videos. While you are freshly tuned into this new topic, ❏ doing the self-help exercises will be easier and the whole topic should remain at the forefront of your mind. ❏

In the following chapters, we will look at:

1. The design and structure of the foot and why it's so important. ❏
2. How your healing rate is affected and why even a small wound can deteriorate quickly. ❏
3. How people with diabetes are more at risk of getting infections and are less likely to be able to fight them off. ❏
4. How our blood vessels can be affected by diabetes, the passage of time and other diseases. ❏
5. How our bodies communicate through the nervous system and the damaging effect that diabetes can have. Too often, people with diabetes are unaware of the imminent danger facing them. ❏

6. Sometimes, however well defended we are, surprises can take us off guard. This chapter is not exhaustive but will give examples you can learn from of where other people have been caught off guard. ❏

7. Finally we will wrap up this section with a chapter of self-help advice so that you can learn how best to minimise your risk. ❏

Key learning.

Know why your feet are important.

Exercise: get into the sweet spot

What I want you to do right now is revisit the tick boxes in this chapter and answer the questions or complete the statements below.

1. What is the most important thing that you have learned in this chapter?

....

....

....

....

2. Which main risk factor have you become aware of?

....

....

....

....

3. The one big thing I am going to start/stop doing is

....

....

....

....

If you need to break that down into several steps, please go ahead and note them below. Make sure to add the date by which you intend to achieve each of those steps.

....

....

....

....

Chapter 7:
Foot structure and deformity.

When I was in my early 20s I bought my dream car, a Ford Capri Mk 3. I could see myself driving around in it like Bodie from the hit TV series of the time *The Professionals*. Shortly afterwards I was involved in a crash which was deemed to be my fault (not because I was driving like Bodie) and the car was written off by the insurance company. To add insult to injury I'd only covered it with third-party insurance so I didn't get a penny for it. In fact I had to pay back the bank loan for another three years. Ouch! Still I had enjoyed the car so I set about looking for another older and cheaper version.

The first one, although newer, had been parked on a garage forecourt under a tree and didn't look as pristine as this older and cheaper vehicle with glossy black paint. It was a Mk 1 and was about 10 years older. It had done many times over the mileage of the other one but beggars can't be choosers so after my basic checks on tyres, oil, brake fluid, the vitally important music system, and having taken a test drive, I handed over the asking price. All seemed in good order, two months tax and 10 months MOT and even half a tank of petrol.

It wasn't long afterwards that I noticed the paint beginning to bubble in several places and it soon became apparent that a lot of filler had been used to patch it up. It went well until one day going down the motorway the exhaust fell off leaving what must have been a magnificent trail of sparks behind me until I could pull over safely. This mishap was followed by the cam belt going and then the suspension. Finally after failing its MOT the following year it was scrapped.

That beautiful machine which had looked so wonderful to the unprofessional eye was in fact a death trap. It seemed so obvious when it was pointed out to me by an expert. This is just one example of how things can appear to be okay to the uninitiated, while trained eyes would quickly spot serious problems that could escalate and be dangerous even to the point of death.

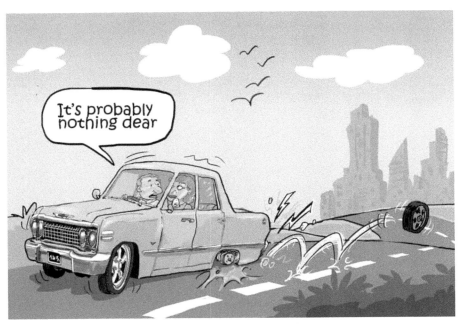

But then again it may be!

Why do we look to the professional to check our second hand car before we buy it or have those annual MOT check-ups or services every 6000 miles? Surely because we have been made aware of their importance and that the mechanic is an expert who can see things we can't.

It never ceases to amaze me how many people never think about getting their feet checked even when they have a problem. Putting up with problems or trying to fix it yourself usually causes much bigger issues later on especially in a person with diabetes. As with the dangers of buying an unchecked second-hand car, it could lead to a serious inability to perform and, possibly, a premature death.

Are you an expert in feet? If not, isn't it time you went to see one?

Imagine for a minute that the car you are thinking of buying has a serious defect that you are oblivious to. At what point would you like to become aware of it? After you've handed over the cash or after you've had the crash? Both of these options are way too late.

Earlier I used the analogy of the fort with its strong walls being vital to its success as a defensive stronghold. While on holiday last year we visited Aberystwyth Castle or what's left of it. Yes it may be ruined today, yet it served its purpose for many years. As I stood next to the walls I marvelled at just how thick they were. But although we may appreciate the finished building, we rarely pay any attention to the months of work preparing the all-important foundations.

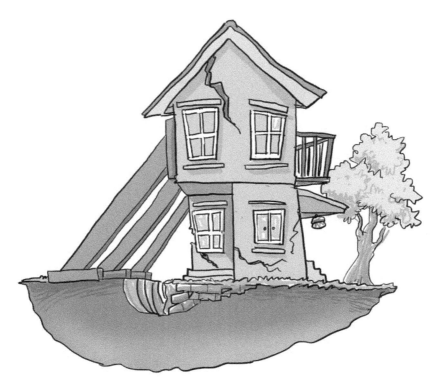

Just as poor foundations can cause a house to crack higher up, so too your feet can cause problems higher up in your body.

Take the famous Petronas Twin Towers of Kuala Lumpur, where the site had to be relocated by 200 feet after tests showed the bedrock was unstable. In fact the original construction site effectively sat on the edge of an underground cliff. Because of the depth of the bedrock and weight that was going to be supported the buildings were built on the world's deepest foundations consisting of 104 concrete piles, ranging from 60 to 114 metres deep (197 to 374 ft) and a 15 ft deep concrete raft consisting of 470,000 cubic feet of concrete for each tower. The foundations themselves took 12 months to complete.

The architects realised the importance of the strength of the foundations for the Petronas towers. Likewise you need to realise that your feet are vitally important to your wellbeing. This is true for all of ❑ us and all the more so as someone living with diabetes.

Broadly speaking the main effects of the foot structure are:

- Postural misalignments leading to arthritic changes and mechanical failure in turn leading to a lack of mobility which results in increased weight over time and in particular higher blood sugars.
- Deformity within the foot which can lead to pressure points that in turn are more at risk of developing sores – especially important in people with diabetes.

Here follows some of the classic deformities that we see on a daily basis and that are most likely to present in your feet later on in life.

Effects of Hallux limitus on the big toe

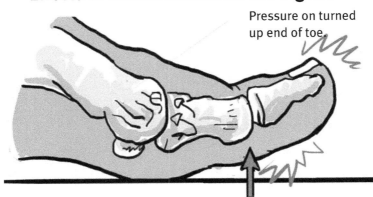

Pressure on turned up end of toe.

Increased pressure causing callus and potentially ulceration under big toe.

- Hammer toes.
- Claw toes.
- Retracted toes.
- Mallet toes.
- Bunions.
- Tailor's bunion.
- Hallux limitus/rigidus.

Primary   **Secondary**   **Tertiary**

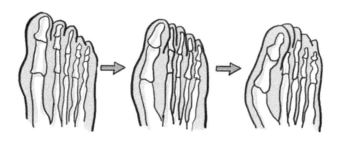

3 stages of bunion development

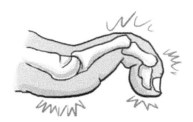

Claw toe

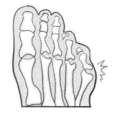

Tailor's bunion

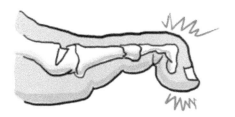

Mallet toe

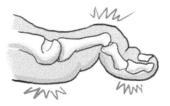

Hammer toe

Case Study

A few months back Maria, a lady with diabetes, was referred to me because her knee pain was affecting her ability to walk. She was a pleasant lady of average build who had always kept active, gardening, walking her dogs and up until about a year ago jogging. A couple of years ago her knee had started to give her some aggro and had caused her to decrease her exercise. She had resigned herself to the fact that at 52 she was getting older and was not meant to be running any more.

Things had deteriorated so much over the preceding eight months that it was an ordeal walking her dogs, which now often only got a run in her back garden. She felt pretty depressed about this and to add insult to injury her Hb1ac blood test was up. Her GP was sure this was because of the lack of exercise and advised swimming which she wasn't keen on never having been a strong swimmer. Thankfully he also understood the potential benefit that podiatry may be able to offer and so referred her to our practice.

On examination I saw that as she walked her feet were collapsing down in such a way that they had probably caused her knee problem over the years and were likely to be aggravating the problem now.

I gave her my usual spiel about how it would have been better to have caught it earlier and that it may be too far gone to help much now. But I was quietly confident from previous experience of this common problem that the exercises and orthotic insoles I would prescribe could make a difference not only to her pain but also her enjoyment of life (and her dogs' enjoyment of life) and therefore also her blood glucose control.

Maria, like many other people, was helped by the use of orthotics and is now able to enjoy walking her dogs. I await her next three monthly blood test to confirm whether her Hb1ac improves as expected with her increased activity. It still remains a fact that earlier intervention is best so if you have never been assessed get along to your local podiatrist and at least have them watch the way you walk. This type of appointment would be called gait analysis and, if necessary, it will be followed by a thorough biomechanical examination of your lower limbs which will give the podiatrist the information they need to be able to prescribe insoles specifically suitable for your feet.

A poor foot structure can lead to all of the following:

1. Poor posture. You are probably not aware that your foot structure can have an impact all the way up your body and that it affects the way you walk and your whole posture. When addressing it with special insoles called functional orthotics it is not uncommon for people to report that their shoulder or neck problem resolves or even that their jaw has stopped clicking. Many of the lower back problems affecting people's lifestyles have the root of their problem in the foot structure. Take a look at the videos on

The effects of Foot pronation on posture

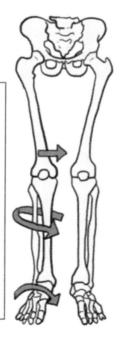
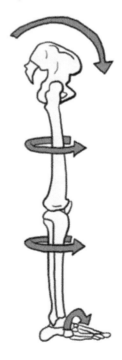

Diagram to show how when the right foot pronates (i.e: rolls down) the whole leg will rotate inwards and the pelvis will tilt anteriorly (towards the front)
If a foot is abnormally pronating it follows that the knees and hips can be affected as well as extra strain put on the lower back

www.undefeeted.org and see how the foot affects the knee ❏ for example. The same can be said for the hip position causing the foot to do strange things and often a leg length difference can cause one foot to behave very differently to the other. I have come to believe that poor posture is to blame for many of our daily complaints and yes of course sometimes it's poor seated posture at a computer desk which should also be addressed; but the foot's structure affecting the way we walk is a major contributing factor that is often overlooked. ❏

In the short-term poor posture will usually present as muscle fatigue, tightness or overuse, trapped nerves or inflamed nerves such as in sciatica. All of these can affect your ability to exercise and therefore maintain good blood glucose control. ❏

2. **Decreased activity.** With non diabetics as well as people with diabetes inactivity usually sets up a vicious cycle of events. Firstly let's consider a person's journey from not having diabetes to developing type 2 later in ❏ life. Let's not forget that approximately 85% of diabetes cases are type 2 and diagnosis comes after years of living without it.

Case Study

Janet was a charming lady and happily married with two children, she had held down a good position as a staff nurse at her local hospital for many years. The trouble was that her weight had fluctuated wildly as she went on every fad diet going. She just couldn't keep the weight off and every January she realised that she was a little heavier. By the time I met her she had given up on the fight and accepted it as her lot. She had been referred to me as she had recently been diagnosed with type 2 diabetes. Additionally she took medication for high blood pressure and high cholesterol and had been informed by her doctor that she really must help herself by losing some of her excess weight.

She so badly needed to exercise to get the positive calorie balance required for her to lose weight. The problem was she had given exercise her best but her knees just wouldn't let her do it. She told me how every morning as she got up she was reminded of her

---

predicament and age not by pain, which generally came on later in the day when she had been on her feet for a while, but by the incredible stiffness she felt.

"I used to be in my school's cross-country team. I'd never have thought I'd end up like this," she said.

Little did she know that her feet were actually the cause of her knee pain and that addressing their structure would allow her to participate in much more exercise and lose the weight which would in turn allow her blood pressure and cholesterol levels to fall as well as helping reduce her blood glucose levels.

In fact it dawned on her that those little supports called orthotics (which she had been advised to get years before) could have improved the quality of her life and her general health.

Less activity and increased weight can have a knock on effect on wear on joints and lead to swelling of the feet and further pressure points. So you get a cycle of events...

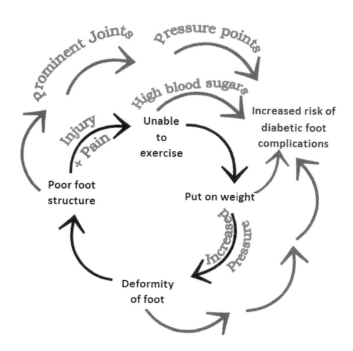

3. **Depression.** For many people every day starts in a similar way to Janet's; they wake up and realise that they can't do as much as they used to. ❑ Obviously there can be many socio-economic reasons contributing to their overall feelings, but it certainly won't make anyone feel any happier knowing they can't do what they used to or indeed what they need to do. In my role as a podiatrist it is overwhelmingly rewarding to hear from clients who no longer suffer pain and who feel their whole life has become brighter because they have been able to get back to doing things they enjoy.

4. **Blood sugar levels.** Your foot structure can affect your blood sugar levels. This can happen in two ways. Firstly by pain causing ❑ decreased activity which will affect you over the long-term. Secondly poor foot structure can lead to a wound that then gets infected. Then as the body fights the infection your blood sugars go all over the place.

5. **Blood pressure.** This will increase as a direct consequence of too little exercise and so anything causing a person to stop exercising, ❑ such as foot, knee or other pain can lead to inactivity and consequently to increased blood pressure.

6. **Heart disease and PAD.** Heart attacks and strokes are often pinpointed as the cause of death even though the underlying ❑ contributory causative factor may have been a sedentary life. (By the way diabetes also massively increases the risk of these.)

7. Continuing your everyday life with **muscles working out of synch** can mean that in the long run **muscles become weak and/ or tight.** ❑

8. Additionally abnormal stresses on the joints can lead to wear and tear on the joint surfaces and deterioration of the cartilage that forms the smooth surface on which the bones articulate together. Ultimately ❑ the bone itself can become eroded. The abnormal alignment of the joints can also cause extra pressure on the bones which can respond by laying down more bone as in the case of the top surfaces of the big toe joint or the back of the heel. The ligaments can also be affected if they are in a constant state of increased strain.

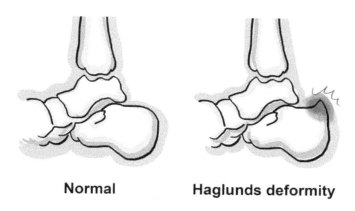

Normal   **Haglunds deformity**

Excessive pressure on the heel bone causing extra bone to be formed.

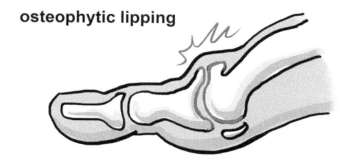

osteophytic lipping

A common condition where jamming of the joint at the base of the big toe causes extra bone to form leading to loss of movement, pain and deformity.

Some of the common foot deformities (in addition to those on page 87) are shown on the previous page. These develop over time as a result of abnormal stresses on the foot either by abnormal function causing muscles to pull out of alignment or by tight shoes or a combination of both.

Tell tale signs

Certain things should alert you to problems with your foot structure.

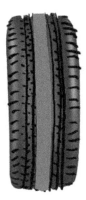 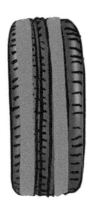 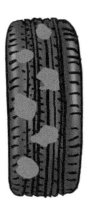 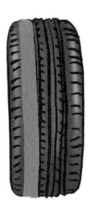

Just as your car tyres can tell you something is wrong, so too your shoes can warn you your foot is not working properly.

The simplest check doesn't even involve you looking at your feet.

Just as a good mechanic can read the warning signs of uneven wear on the tyres of a car, your shoes will often give an indication of how your foot is working.

If you're at home, take your shoes off right now and check the wear marks on them. If you're not at home, set an alarm on your phone or write a note to remind you to do this on your return.

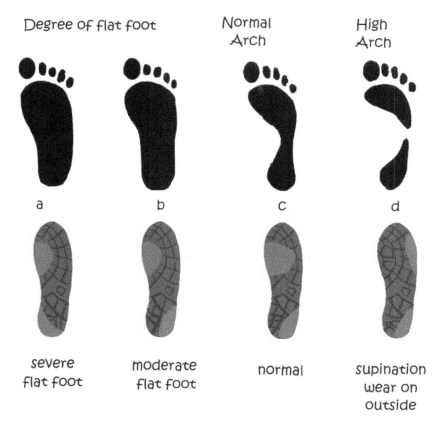

Degree of flat foot | Normal Arch | High Arch

a   b   c   d

severe flat foot   moderate flat foot   normal   supination wear on outside

- Is the wear more on one side of the heel than the other?
- Is it on the outside edge of the forefoot or the inside?
- Is the left more worn than the right?
- Are the uppers leaning to one side or another?
- Do they show scuff marks for example on the inside of the heels or are there prominent bulges over a bunion, hammer toe or where the big toe nail turns up?

A podiatrist will give you the professional view on how normally your shoes are wearing.

Next take your socks off. Do they wear out unevenly? Are they particularly sweaty and if so do they smell, or are they full of dry skin? I recently treated a gentleman with diabetes who came to me because he'd noticed when he took his socks off at the end of the day they were damp above his big toe nail. On further investigation

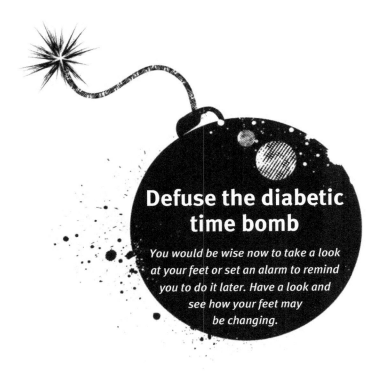

it was found that his big toe nails had got so thick that the pressure on the nail bed had caused it to ulcerate. If he hadn't noticed and taken action then those ulcers could easily have become infected and possibly led to gangrene, amputation and even a premature death. ❏

All those dire consequences because of a toe nail that needed thinning down! A small problem that can be taken care of in one simple podiatry appointment can so easily become a major issue over time.

Defuse the diabetic time bomb

You would be wise now to take a look at your feet or set an alarm to remind you to do it later. Have a look and see how your feet may be changing.

Now you're looking at your feet, what can you see? (If you can't see them then get a loved one to check them for you). If you are alone and can't see too well then use a mirror or your phone or camera to ❏ take pictures so you can inspect them properly. If anything concerns you go and see your podiatrist or at the very least send a photo to them asking for their opinion. (Bear in mind that sometimes it is not easy to diagnose and advise from just a photo).

Look for any of the following:

- Open wounds.
- Red prominences.
- Inflamed areas.
- Blisters.
- Hard skin including corns or verrucae.
- Are there any cracks particularly in the heels?
- Thickened nails or curling nails.
- Discolouration of the nails.
- Athletes foot especially between the toes.
- Dark skin areas.
- Moles – and have they changed?
- Swollen areas.
- Deformities. Some examples are bunions, claw toes, hammer toes, mallet toes, retracted toes, tailor's bunions, prominent metatarsal heads, hyper extended big toe joint, bony deposits called osteophytic lipping over the big toe joint (see the images on pages 87 and 93), trigger toe.

If you find any of these then either go and train as a podiatrist or go and see one for their professional opinion. It is much better to be told it's nothing serious and address it than to wait until it progresses and becomes something limb-threatening.

Different types of foot.

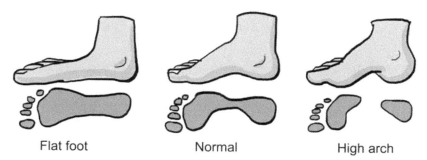

Flat foot   Normal   High arch

Here's one more check that you can do for yourself. If your bathroom floor is tiled, next time you get out of the bath see what footprint you leave on the floor. Does the arch flatten out as in the flat foot diagram on the left or is there little pressure in the middle of the foot like the high arched foot on the right? Perhaps it is relatively normal as in the middle example. Beware though; if it looks normal don't be lulled in to a false sense of security, this is not the only way that your foot structure can let you down. See the vidos on **www.undefeeted.org** for more information.

What can be done?

Generally a poor foot structure will need to be addressed either with better shoes or, more often, with special insoles and occasionally with surgery, or a combination of the above. The longer the problem is left the more likely that the benefits of treatment will be limited.

Early intervention is always best even if the outcome is merely advice on how to monitor a particular issue. I believe that every child should have three foot checks before their 18th birthday. This would allow them to have any obvious defects noted and addressed if appropriate. It may seem excessive at first but please consider that an estimated 70-80% of us inherit an abnormal foot structure and that by the age of 18, those feet will probably have carried us at least once around the world.

Compare the three visits I am suggesting to the 32 times you are recommended to take your child to the dentist between the ages of two and 18. Why neglect your kids' feet? Get them checked too and give your children a good foundation for their future wellbeing.

At this stage in life it is important to be aware of the damage that can be done by not allowing the foot to function normally. As podiatrists we aim to address the abnormal function taking place as a result of poor foot structure. This can sometimes be in the form of insoles or even single heel raises to address a leg length difference.

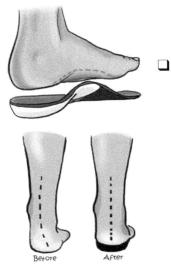

Before   After

Right foot

Sometimes we just recommend exercises to allow the muscles to catch up with the bones during growth and so alleviate growing pains.

As a person grows older there is often resultant deformity and secondary problems in the form of arthritic changes in the feet, knees and hips. As such it often becomes less possible to address the function of the feet and orthotics are frequently prescribed to accommodate rather than change the function. As a general rule an orthotic will wherever possible aim to improve the function of the feet and prevent further deterioration.

Sadly we often don't see people until time has done its dirty work on their feet, giving them bunions, hammer and claw toes or dropped arches. Alongside accommodative orthotics a person may be advised to get their shoes stretched or altered. Later still – and if the deformity has become too much – a person may have no choice but to get bespoke hospital surgical shoes which tend to be very bulky and not very attractive.

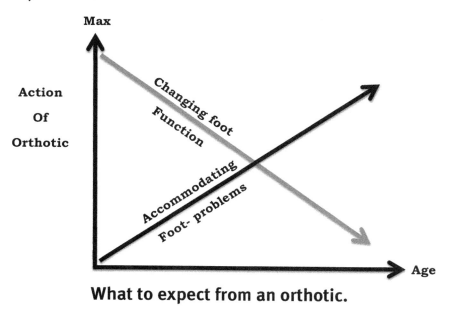

What to expect from an orthotic.

Exercise: get into the sweet spot

Take a look at the tick boxes in this chapter and answer the questions or complete the statements below.

1. What is the most important thing that you have learned in this chapter?

....

....

....

....

2. Which main risk factor have you become aware of?

....

....

....

....

3. The one big thing I am going to start/stop doing is

....

....

....

....

If you need to break that down into several steps, please go ahead and note them below. Make sure to add the date by which you intend to achieve each of those steps.

....

....

....

....

Chapter 8:
Healing rate.

As the largest organ of the body, the human skin has to protect against puncture wounds, cuts, grazes and infections. It is the body's first line of defence. The truth is we tend to take it for granted and don't appreciate how amazing it is especially in repairing itself. Most of us probably give the incredible regenerative powers of the skin little thought, just putting a plaster on when we cut ourselves. We assume it will heal.

I was once told that the word assume actually means 'make an ASS out of U and ME' and this has become a mantra for me in life generally.

This is particularly important for you as someone with diabetes. You cannot just assume a wound, however small, will heal. In fact it is ❏ better to assume it won't and give it all the help you can.

As wound healing is complex, I am only going to give you a basic outline of how healing takes place in a normal non diabetic foot and impress upon you the fact that it doesn't happen as well in the foot of a person with diabetes. ❏

First let me introduce you to James. James is a 10-year-old in perfect health. He has everything going for him with regards to good healing of the numerous wounds he is likely to incur as a boy of that age.

As soon as James cuts himself, the wound undergoes numerous complex processses which together allow the wound to heal. These can largely be grouped into three phases that happen in the following order (although one phase will overlap with another).

1. Inflammatory phase: aims to stop blood loss and prevent infection.
2. Repair phase: aims to restore normal function to that skin.
3. Remodelling phase: aims to restore normal function, structure and appearance to that skin.

The inflammatory phase ❏

This should begin as soon as you cut yourself .Your body has two main objectives: to stop any bleeding and to prevent or kill any infection. Initially the local blood vessels undergo vasoconstriction (which means they contract) making them narrower so you lose less blood. At the same time a temporary mesh (fibrin protein) forms which helps with the clotting process by allowing platelets in your blood to attach to it. This prevents further bleeding.

Then the blood vessels vasodilate (which means they widen) allowing more blood to get to the wound to help repair it. Often there is localised swelling at the wound as fluid containing inflammatory cells and proteins enters the area aiming to give a good healthy inflammatory response. This fluid contains special inflammatory cells called neutrophils and macrophages whose job it is to go around the wound and eat up any debris or bacteria, breaking them down into less harmful smaller bits which the body can get rid of.

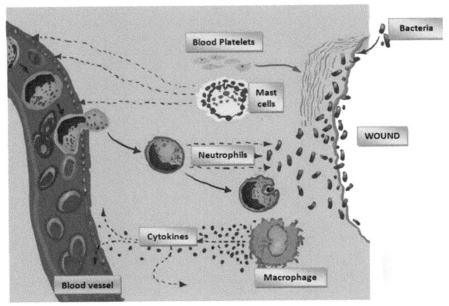

Normal process of wound healing

Love them or hate them many of you will have heard of the 1960s TV series called Thunderbirds. I like to think of the inflammatory cells as Thunderbirds. Neutrophils travel around in your blood waiting for an alarm bell and as soon as the skin is wounded they are alerted. I will call them Thunderbirds 1. Once alerted, they rush to the site, exit the blood vessel and launch into the hostile environment of the wound where they attack any debris or bacteria. This takes place in the first few hours following the injury.

Following close behind are the Thunderbirds 2 – the macrophages which remain in the wound for days or weeks doing the clean-up operation on any remaining debris or infection.

The proliferative stage ❏

The next stage is when the body closes and fills up the wound and this begins from a few days after the initial injury and can last a few weeks. Thunderbirds 3 are called into action in the form of fibroblasts and together with the macrophages help form another more complex but still temporary tissue matrix called granulation tissue. This replaces the temporary fibrin mesh. New blood vessels are formed and a process called epithelialisation begins where new cells from the edges of the wound multiply to fill the gap whilst the fibroblasts help by pulling the matrix together, thus causing the wound to contract and close.

The remodelling stage ❏

This takes place weeks and months after the initial wound. The matrix and its cellular content mature to become more and more like normal skin. Eventually the healed tissue will be as healthy as it was before, although in some cases it heals with scar tissue within it. Either way the body has fulfilled its primary function of restoring a barrier for protection from infection and usually restoring normal function.

In an ideal situation this is how your body will heal from wounds both small and large. However diabetes is not an ideal situation and I could write pages on how it affects wound healing, but then you'd probably close the book and never open it again. The important thing for you to grasp is that wound healing deteriorates in someone with diabetes. There is plenty of detailed information online if you wish to ❏ research it in more depth.

The above mentioned mechanisms of healing are in themselves associated with other factors discussed in this part of the book. There are usually a number of factors that together form the worst environment for healing to take place. These factors are

- High blood glucose levels.
- Neuropathy.
- Peripheral arterial disease.
- Deformity.
- Swelling.
- Inactivity.
- Infection.

Other factors such as obesity, stress, depression, and anxiety can also hinder healing and unfortunately they often coexist with diabetes. ❏

These factors also have a detrimental effect on our healing rate:

- Smoking. ❏
- Poor diet.
- Alcohol and drug misuse. ❏
- Some medications.
- Our environment, such as how warm we keep our house.

Prevention is better than cure.

Prevention is always better than cure in diabetic wound care. Most wounds can be prevented if you take steps to minimise risk.

Common causes of wounds and how to prevent them:

1. Tight shoes. Buy shoes at the end of the day (your feet are likely ❏ to be a bit swollen then) and see if you can persuade the shop to let you wear them at home for a while. Carefully monitor for any discomfort, especially any signs of pressure or rubbing. Remember that nice pair you last wore two years ago may not be the right fit for you now, so try them on the day before you plan to wear them.

A good friend of mine loves his Gucci shoes but they kill his little toe every time he wears them. That's not because there is anything wrong with the shoe, it's just that either his foot shape, size or foot function is not suited to that particular design. If, like him, you have a favourite pair of shoes that hurt your feet, then throw them away or recycle them. If you can't bear to do that straightaway, ❏ check to see if a cobbler or your podiatrist can stretch the leather over the tight spot. ❏

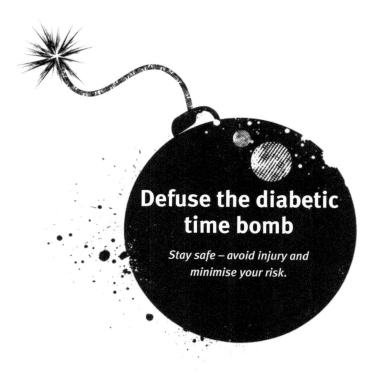

Defuse the diabetic time bomb

Stay safe – avoid injury and minimise your risk.

2. **Loose shoes.** Shoes can become loose as they get worn and can do as much damage as ones that are too tight. Make sure you wear a ❏ shoe with a fastening and don't just slip them on. Insoles can also help create a snugger fit. Please see the section on footwear choices in Part Three. ❏

3. Foreign body (i.e. glass or even a dog hair). Puncture wounds are dangerous because as the foreign body enters your flesh it can carry bacteria with it and even when it is removed it leaves behind a little ❑ culture of bugs in your tissues which can then secretly multiply and spread the infection even into the bone.

4. Blister. A blister can be caused by new activities, new shoes or a foot that is functioning abnormally because of a bad structure. ❑

5. Callus and corns are very common and if maintained regularly and offloaded with padding or insoles should not pose a problem. ❑ You would be wise to ask your podiatrist why they are forming as you may be able to have bespoke insoles prescribed which will allow the foot to behave more normally and change the areas of high pressure and friction that causes the hard skin. ❑

6. Cracked skin. Dry hard skin will crack as it is less supple and these cracks can worsen until they reach the dermis and become open wounds. The hard skin must be professionally removed and the ❑ skin kept hydrated for the best chance of the fissure totally healing up. However that place will always be prone to cracking so you must maintain it as described in the self-help pages in Part Three. ❑

7. Thickened nails. Thickened nails can be caused by one-off traumatic events, gradual repetitive trauma over a number of years, and fungal infection. Once thick they are likely to have pressure on them from footwear and can ulcerate under the nail leading to infection. ❑

8. Athletes foot. This fungal infection is not dangerous in itself but, as the skin can break, it is easy for a secondary bacterial infection to take hold. ❑

9. Self treatments such as DIY treatments, picking at nails or callus or simply cutting nails too short. ❑

10. Pressure sores from inactivity or from deformity. ❑

11. Burns can blister and break open causing a wound. ❑

12. Chilling can lead to death of the superficial tissues which can then break open and ulcerate. ❑

13. Ingrowing toe nails. A toe nail can either curl to form an involuted shape or have a sharp corner left from poor nail cutting. Both of ❏ these scenarios can lead to a break in the skin and subsequently a wound that is open to infection.

Key learnings to keep you in the sweet spot:

1. Be aware that injuries may not heal as easily.
2. Get professional advice. You may need a specialist wound dressing rather than a simple plaster.
3. Think risk assessment before gardening, doing diy jobs etc. Minimise the risk of injury.

Exercise: get into the sweet spot.

It's time to look at the tick boxes in this chapter and answer the questions or complete the statements below.

1. What is the most important thing that you have learned in this chapter?

....

....

....

....

2. Which main risk factor have you become aware of?

....

....

....

....

3. The one big thing I am going to start/stop doing is

....

....

....

....

If you need to break that down into several steps, please go ahead and note them below. Make sure to add the date by which you intend to achieve each of those steps.

....

....

....

....

Chapter 9:
Circulation.

Two major complications of diabetes are associated with its affects on your circulation firstly on your major arteries and secondly on your much smaller capillaries. Both of these are vitally important to your health as they enable your life-giving blood to circulate and reach your cells.

I am often reminded of a journey I took several years ago. There was nothing special about it, I knew it well as I travelled the length of the M11 twice a week to provide consultations for my patients in the Cambridge area. Today however was different even though I was taking the same route. One decision was going to change my entire day. Rather than listening to the radio as usual, I was going to play a new CD from my favourite artist. The first part of the journey across South London was uneventful and I didn't think anything of the slightly heavier amount of traffic, but then as I ground to a halt in Greenwich, I realised something was wrong.

I decided it was time to give Meatloaf a break and switched over to the radio to hear the travel news. I learned there had been an accident in the Blackwall Tunnel and the whole of south-east London was in gridlock.

I really wished I'd turned on the radio earlier! If I'd known sooner I could have gone a different way. As it was, two hours later I had hardly moved. Eventually I crawled home having earned nothing that day and I had to sacrifice my day off the following week so I could see my patients.

I am not the first to equate the road system with our circulation; terms such as main arterial route and bypass are often used. Living in London we are acutely aware of the need to keep traffic flowing and the dire consequences of a blockage in the road system.

A city's success relies in part on having an efficient transport system to get people around and deliveries of goods in. Imagine a city with no way of getting its waste picked up and out of the way. So too the body has a complex network of arteries and capillaries transporting nutrients, oxygen, white blood cells and medicines to every living cell and veins transporting waste products away. And our feet are the ❏ furthest part of the body from the main distributor, the heart. ❏

Normal   **Early Atherosclerosis**   **Severe Atherosclerosis**

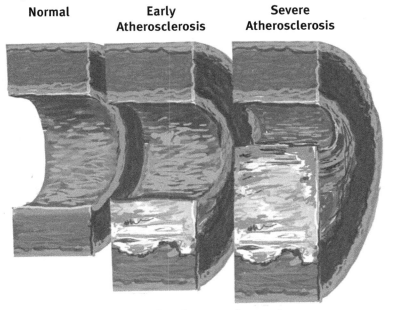

Degrees of Atherosclerosis

Even in non diabetics arteries will be affected by time, a high fat ❏ diet, smoking, the side effects of some drugs and lack of exercise, as well as by other medical conditions. When a person becomes diabetic they become more likely to develop circulatory complications in the big arteries (macrovascular disease) which can lead to problems such ❏ as myocardial infarction (cardiac arrest), cerebrovascular accident (stroke) and there is also a heightened risk to the peripheral arteries leading to ulceration and gangrene with possible loss of limb. As the arteries to the feet are the longest ones in the body these changes will ❏ show up earliest and have the most dramatic effect.

Arteries don't usually show on an x-ray but when they have become hardened with calcium deposits, as they do in some people with diabetes, they may. Another complication is that the person may be unaware of these problems if they suffer with the common diabetic ❏ complication of neuropathy meaning they could have a silent myocardial infarction (heart attack with no pain associated with it).

When the peripheral arteries become affected in a non diabetic it is called peripheral arterial disease (PAD) and the person will often be alerted to the problem by a condition called intermittent claudication. ❏ This happens when the circulation deteriorates to the point that the muscles in the lower leg and sometimes the thigh don't get enough oxygen and painful cramps set in after walking even a short distance. Resting will allow them to recover and so the person sets off again only to experience the same pain further down the road. This person is likely to seek help because of the discomfort; as a person with diabetes you may have the same level of PAD but be unaware of it. ❏

If the PAD becomes more severe the non diabetic will usually complain of pain even when at rest at night-time. This is called rest ❏ pain and if the intermittent claudication hasn't sent them to their GP yet then this will. In a person who has diabetes with neuropathy this can also go unnoticed as they can't feel anything wrong. It's a bit ❏ like me not knowing there was a problem ahead at Blackwall Tunnel because I hadn't heard the travel news.

That problem started with an accident which caused a narrowing of the main arterial route allowing fewer cars through and which became blocked as the emergency services attended so that no cars were able to pass. This can be equated to macrovascular disease and its effects. Later the traffic backed up in the smaller roads feeding ❏ into the main ones and the whole area became gridlocked. This can be likened to microvascular disease where the smallest blood vessels ❏ in the body become affected.

STAGE 1

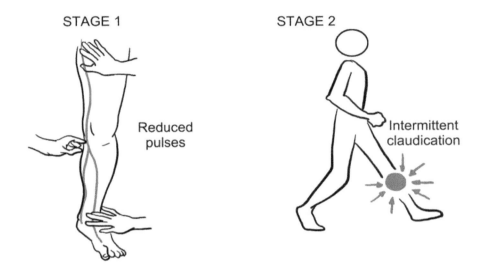

Reduced
pulses

STAGE 2

Intermittent
claudication

STAGE 3

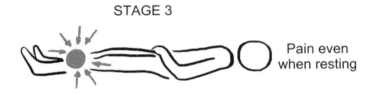

Pain even
when resting

STAGE 4

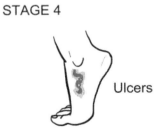

Ulcers

The small blood vessels supply:

- The eyes. If affected this can lead to retinopathy and therefore ❏ blindness.
- The kidneys. If affected it can lead to nephropathy and ultimately renal failure requiring regular dialysis. ❏
- The sensory, autonomic, and motor nerves. (See Chapter 10). ❏

The dangers of poor circulation

Ischemia (inadequate blood supply) can have numerous consequences on the feet:

- Chronic ischemia (gradual long-term effects). ❏
- Thinner and weaker skin more prone to damage. ❏
- Less nutrition and oxygen is delivered to the cells. ❏
- Waste is not removed as efficiently. ❏
- Decreased healing of damaged tissues due to lack of oxygen and ❏ nutrients.
- Decreased ability to fight infection as white blood cells are not ❏ able to get there.
- Neuropathy: because their feet aren't warning them people tend ❏ to walk more. The more pressure on their feet the longer the blood is squeezed out of the areas of high pressure leading to hard skin and ulcers.
- Decreased temperature and formation of areas of chilling. ❏
- Cracked dry heels. ❏
- Poorer vision. ❏

Acute ischemia

Sometimes an acute attack of ischemia can present and needs to be addressed as a clinical emergency. With a diabetic there may be reduced pain or even no pain at all. Signs to watch out for are: ❑

- Sudden change to normality in one lower limb (compare the right and left leg).
- Limb becomes cold further down from the blockage.
- Change in colour to a mottled effect.
- Pale distal (far end) of the leg.
- Painful (may not be so in a person with diabetes).
- If you have a digital infrared thermometer you are likely to find a temperature gradient from the shin to the end of the big toe on the affected side with the toe being lower due to the lack of blood supply.

If a non diabetic with this type of problem is not treated quickly then they may well lose the limb. Early intervention is even more ❑ important for a person with diabetes. Early diagnosis and subsequent speedy treatment is essential if the foot or leg is to be saved. Treatment may include the need for a bypass, angioplasty or the use of longer term anticoagulants.

What to keep an eye open for.

There are certain things you can keep an eye on yourself but the earlier you get professional help the better. Getting help once you are aware of a problem is too late. The best and most effective time to get help is before you are aware of any problems and thus self observation should never be allowed to replace regular professional assessment. ❑

Signs to observe:

1. Feet becoming colder than normal so comparing both feet can be helpful. (If infection is present the temperature may be elevated). ❑
2. Loss of hair. ❑
3. Thin shiny skin. ❑
4. Dry skin. ❑

5. Swollen feet/ankles (may indicate heart or kidney problems). ❑
6. Colour changes to the extremities and areas of high pressure such ❑ as ends of toes, bunions and the metatarsal heads, especially in cold weather.
7. Sudden onset of cold. ❑

If we're not told about the blocked tunnel ahead by those in the know, such as the police, we gradually become aware of it when we grind to a halt. If we're alerted to the problem in advance we can choose an alternative route.

Even before becoming diabetic, circulatory changes take place because of age or other diseases. Unfortunately this usually happens without us being aware and it's why peripheral arterial disease is often referred to as the silent killer. ❑

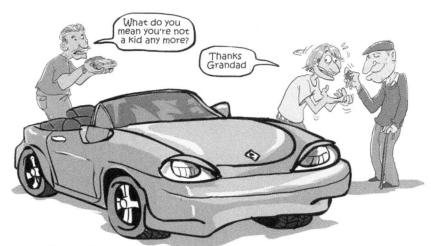

Sometimes when you live with them every day you just don't notice the changes!

Its effects are a bit like watching the kids grow up. If you're living with your kids you are less likely to notice the changes than if you are a ❑ relative who only sees them a couple of times a year.

For 'relative' read 'podiatrist' who will see your feet less often than you do and so, together with specialised knowledge, they are more ❑ likely to pick up subtle changes in the wellbeing of your lower limbs.

What a podiatrist can tell you about your circulation

Experience and a trained eye will often enable the podiatrist to immediately evaluate the condition of a person's circulation. Additional tools will also be used for a more detailed assessment of their vascular status. This enables a referral to be made if deemed ❏ necessary, or if not, gives some benchmarks to enable a person's condition to be measured over time. Either way it allows the earliest possible intervention to take place either with advice or treatment be it medication or surgery.

Palpation of pulses

1. There are two main pulses in the foot. As the arteries pass down ❏ the legs and into the feet they become narrower. The pulse of each heartbeat should be felt both behind the inside ankle bone and on the top of the foot. ❏

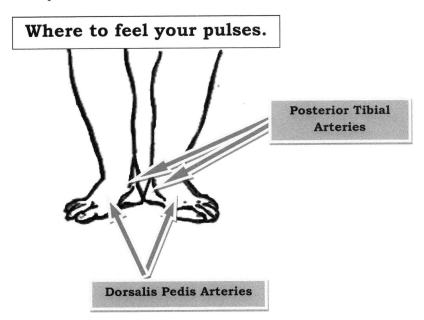

Where to feel your pulses.

Posterior Tibial Arteries

Dorsalis Pedis Arteries

2. Doppler. The pulse doesn't tell us what condition the arteries are in. A simple Doppler uses ultrasound to listen to the blood flow through the arteries. This allows us to detect any major blockages ❏ higher up the leg.

3. An even better Doppler can detect which way the blood is flowing. Most people think the blood flows from the heart to the target area and yes, this is the end result we want, but in fact normal ❏ good blood flow down the arteries occurs in three phases in both directions. These changes in direction can be detected with a bidirectional Doppler and can tell us a lot about the quality of the blood flow. ❏

Normal arterial blood flow is triphasic. Please look at the diagram ❏ opposite where you can compare the common readings. Anything above the line is blood flowing away from the heart whilst below the line is blood flowing back towards the heart.

The first peak indicates blood rushing down as the heart pumps. As the heart relaxes the pressure drops and the blood flows backwards, which shows up on the Doppler trace as a trough below the zero line. The artery walls, if they are still elastic, stretch and recoil squeezing the blood back down the arteries as is evident on the ❏ top diagram where there is a second peak. This serves two main purposes: firstly it encourages better perfusion of blood into the feet and secondly it means the heart doesn't have to work as hard shunting the blood down the arteries.

The bidirectional Doppler can tell us a lot about the state of the arteries in the leg but it should also be remembered that these ❏ arteries being the longest will show up changes earliest. There is a strong likelihood that all the other arteries in the body will also be affected if these are. When I bought one of my Dopplers it arrived from America with a whole pad of insurance referral forms as the insurance companies want to know from this simple test what the risk is of the coronary arteries and arteries in the brain being furred ❏ up. They can then assess the risk of the person having a heart attack or stroke and increase the premium accordingly.

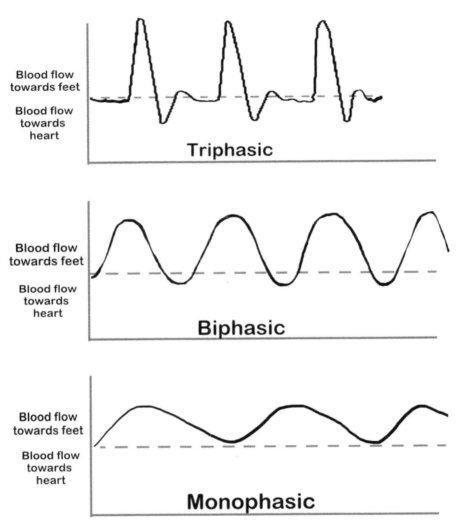

Triphasic

Biphasic

Monophasic

4. ABI test. This is a more in-depth test and its results enable the podiatrist to tell you the extent of PAD's effect on your lower limbs. It is worked out by taking the blood pressure of both arms and ankles and working out the ratio between them. The lower your result the worse your PAD is. Sometimes in a diabetic a deceptively high result can be obtained which is due to the arteries having become hardened with calcium deposits.

5. Toe brachial test. Similar to ABI but involves the use of a special small blood pressure cuff which reads the blood pressure of the vessels in the big toe.

6. Capillary refill time. The time it takes for the blood to come back into the toe after it's squeezed out. This is something you can do at home – simply squeeze the end of your toe gently but firmly, let go and time how long it takes for the colour to come back. Ideally ❑ it should take about three seconds. In my experience it can take a while even in some young healthy people so in the absence of any other negative findings it is not too serious. However it should alert you to the fact that if it takes a long time for the capillaries to fill up whilst your arteries are functioning well then if you allow your arteries to deteriorate (or fur up), it will become even harder for the bloow to fill the capillaries leading to complications both ❑ in healing and in cold weather.

7. **Temperature gradient**. Using the back of your hand or a friend's is a basic way of assessing temperature differences in the leg and foot. In recent years the use of infra red digital thermometers has ❑ made it easy for us to check the temperature of the skin surface and can also be an indicator of poor circulation. The lower leg's

Lower limb temperature and what it can tell us.

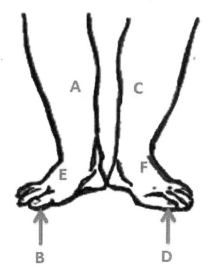

1) Normal temperature at A and C is 28-32*c

2) Ideally A=C and B=D a big difference could indicate a blockage on one side

3) The difference between A and B or C and D should be less than 10*C. If this difference is more than 10*c there is an increased risk of chilling and necrosis.

4) If you suspect an infection or Charcot joint at E, check its temperature and compare it to A and the corresponding place on the opposite foot (in this case F) If E is raised then it is best to suspect a problem and seek professional help.

(For Charcot jt see ch10)

temperature is taken as well as the end of the big toe. We are looking for a small difference – the smaller the better – although there can be a big range of normal readings. What we don't want is a big difference. In my experience, depending on other symptoms, anything over 10 degrees Celsius could be a cause for concern and may need further investigation.

Conversely an elevated temperature can be cause for concern as it may indicate infection, frictional forces or a rare condition called a Charcot joint (see Chapter 10). There is also evidence to suggest that in many cases prior to a breakdown or an ulcer forming, the temperature in that local area may be raised.

Recently it has been shown that if an area of skin is raised in temperature by more than 2.2 degrees centigrade, then there is an increased likelihood of it breaking down into an ulcer in the near future. If a difference like this is noted either compared to the surrounding skin or compared to the same site on the other foot, then a professional opinion should be sought as a matter of urgency.

The final thing we are looking for is a similarity between left and right. If one side is markedly lower than the other it could indicate a blockage in an artery higher up. Conversely if one side is higher a possible infection may be indicated.

8. **Buerger's test**. This is a simple test where the patient lies flat on their back and the podiatrist (or even a friend) raises the person's legs. As they are raised the colour should stay the same if the heart is able to pump strongly enough to get over the effects of gravity. However if the arteries are diseased, then the blood may not be able to make it through and so the feet become pale. The angle the legs make from the couch indicates the degree of ischemia with below 20 degrees indicating severe ischemia. The person then sits up with their feet dangling off the edge of the chair. In the affected leg the blood will take longer to reach the foot and so it will remain paler for longer. Also the colour may go beyond normal becoming more red as the blood vessels attempt to get rid of the toxins and waste products that have built up while there was no blood flow. An example of this test can be watched at **www. undefeeted.org/tv**.

9. Transcutaneous oxygen. This tests the amount of oxygen that is available in the superficial tissue. This is done using an oxometer.

All or some of these tests should be carried out at least once a year by your podiatrist – or more frequently if there are issues that need ❏ monitoring. It allows early detection of potentially limb-threatening diseases. Recent statistics have shown that of the diabetic lower limb amputations in the UK 24% have never had professional care for their feet. The majority of these could probably have been prevented if they had been cared for appropriately. ❏

At the end of your assessment the podiatrist should be able to advise you of your risk if your circulation has deteriorated.

In addition to regular check-ups it is a good idea to get into the habit of checking your own feet every day. People with diabetes are renowned for speedy deterioration leading to avoidable amputation so it makes sense to notice anything unusual quickly and then to take action. Get used to what your feet look like while they are okay (take ❏ photos if necessary) so you will know if they change.

What can be done if your circulation has deteriorated?

I interviewed one of the key people in the prevention of diabetes-related amputation, David Armstrong of the Southern Arizona Limb Salvage Alliance (SALSA). His team has coined the phrase 'Toe or Flow'. This means that anyone attending their clinics with a limb-threatening wound is assessed to identify if the main problem is within the foot and therefore needs the focus of the 'toe team' or if ❏ it is to do with the foot's vascularisation in which case it will need the attention of the 'flow team' led by Dr Joseph Mills. Limbs that previously would have been amputated are now being salvaged as their blood supply is restored and their wound healing improved.

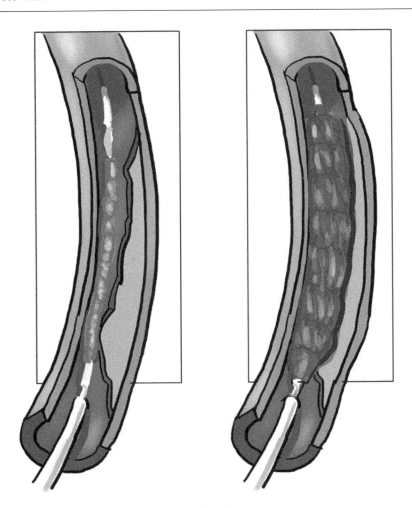

Angioplasty.

There are primarily three types of revascularisation:

1. **Angioplasty.** Most commonly if the blockage is not too bad you may need an angioplasty. This is a minimally invasive procedure involving a thin and flexible tube (a catheter) being inserted into the artery itself via a small incision above the blockage. At the end of this tube is a minute balloon which can be inflated or deflated. This balloon travels down to the blockage in a deflated state and when it arrives it is inflated and deflated pushing the plaque or blockage against the wall of the artery and making more room for the blood to flow again.

2. **Angioplasty with introduction of a stent (a small metal mesh tube).** A stent is inserted during a normal angioplasty to ensure the artery walls in that area don't collapse.

3. **Bypass.** This is a more involved surgical procedure and as the name suggests a surgeon connects either a transplanted blood vessel or an artificial one so that the new vessel allows the blood to pass the original blockage.

4. **Endartectomy.** Occasionally it is possible to surgically remove the blockage.

Promotion of angiogenesis.

Various studies are being carried out that look into the possibility of stimulating the body's own vascular endothelial growth factor to enable the body to grow new blood vessels in the leg.

Your general health and medication, as well as the location and severity of the blockage, will need to be taken into account to determine which procedure will work best for you.

Prevention is better than cure and choosing to eat healthily and exercise daily from today onwards will put you at least risk of developing issues requiring this level of intervention. Choose to be in the sweet spot with your diet and exercise regime and this will help you avoid the sort of deterioration that leads to these interventions.

Exercise: get into the sweet spot.

Please revisit the tick boxes in this chapter and answer the questions or complete the statements below.

1. What is the most important thing that you have learned in this chapter?

....

....

....

....

2. Which main risk factor have you become aware of?

....

....

....

....

3. The one big thing I am going to start/stop doing is

....

....

....

....

If you need to break that down into several steps, please go ahead and note them below. Make sure to add the date by which you intend to achieve each of those steps.

....

....

....

....

Chapter 10:
Neuropathy: how is your dashboard?

Neuropathy is defined as damage or disease affecting the nerves. In the case of diabetes it relates particularly to the peripheral nerves, i.e. the ones at your extremities, the feet and hands in particular.

Case Study

Jack was 72 and overweight at 119 kg and 5 foot 8 inches tall. He usually sported a beaming smile above a double, if not triple, chin. He'd spent all his working life dressed smartly but had taken retirement to extremes and now was mostly seen in baggy trousers and a shirt that had seen better days. If you walked past him in the street you would see him trudging along in a pair of slippers whatever the season. It's an ongoing battle for me to get him to wear more protective footwear. ❏

Being diabetic he sees me for routine care of his nails. Jack was first diagnosed 14 years ago although he'll tell you he may have been diabetic without knowing it for some time. Every year we carry out his diabetic foot assessment, checking his pulses and circulation, which seem still to be adequate, and I routinely check his sensory ❏ nerves. Even though I know he can't feel any of the tests I still do them to drive home to him the fact that he cannot feel and is at risk. ❏

He had come for one of his regular check-ups. My face dropped as I saw a gaping wound in the middle of the sole of his right foot. It still amazes me the extent of injury a person can sustain and yet if they have neuropathy they just won't be aware of it. ❏

I had seen this sort of wound many times but usually where callus had been allowed to build up. I knew Jack usually had very little ❏

---

hard skin and I had only seen him three months before. Taking his slipper I asked him if he was aware of his foot's wound which he assured me he wasn't. I proceeded to pull a half inch carpet tack from the sole of his slipper which was a shock for both of us. Then followed months of dressings, removal of dead skin, antibiotics and visits to the hospital diabetes team. Together we finally got it to heal and to this day Jack can still be seen walking along the high street – and if you were to ask him to lift those trouser legs what would you see but a pair of slippers.

AAAAARGH! It's typical of people with neuropathy not to take advice even though they desperately need it.

Jack now has scarring where the wound was which is always going to be a weak spot and prone to further ulceration if the callus is allowed to build up. Now he has to see me more frequently. ❏

The first time I ever saw Jack and tested his nerves he was unaware that he had lost sensation. **How sure are you that you are okay?** You may still have some sensation but you need to be checked to ❏
see if you have lost some and are now at heightened risk.

The gift of pain

Few of us welcome pain, yet it is a precious gift that has an important underlying purpose. It warns us that something is wrong and ❏
something needs to be done so that there is no further damage done to that part of the body.

I like to think of our bodies as having a dashboard which every day gives us a load of information to keep us safe – for the most part without us being aware of it. We generally live on auto pilot. One of the key warning lights on our dashboard is pain. We often don't take pain seriously enough and put up with it rather than acting on it. I regularly ❏
see new clients who report they first felt pain months or even years before. Can you think of any niggling pains that come and go from time to time? If so then now is the time to get it dealt with rather than waiting for it to become more intense, more constant or more serious. ❏

If you've ever had an old banger of a car like my final Capri you may have found that it drank oil almost faster than petrol and the oil level warning light would regularly light up. You get used to it to the point you don't really notice it. Yet if you bought a brand new car and the oil light switched on what would you do? Most of us would be on the phone booking a professional to check out why it's happening.

Key learnings:
1. Accept you may be at risk.
2. Understand how you may be at risk.
3. Act by putting safeguards into place.

Pain is a gift but unfortunately it often doesn't register on a diabetic person's dashboard. It can deteriorate and become as unreliable as a loose wire and eventually become as useless as a severed wire. Thus although there may be a big problem in your body you may be ❑ oblivious to the danger.

In the absence of having that gift of pain the next best thing is the gift of knowledge of what to look for and when to look for it (so make ❑ sure to keep ticking those boxes and doing the sweet spot exercises). More than any of the others, this chapter is the one where you really need to understand the risks associated with this aspect of diabetes, comprehend how you may be at risk, and put an action plan in place ❑ and into practice without delay. This chapter will hopefully convey to you the importance of putting a system in place to firstly become aware of your need and then to address that need.

How diabetes affects the nerves

The main cause of diabetic neuropathy is lack of nutrition getting to the nerves from the small blood vessels serving them. Thus if we can help the blood vessels stay healthy, the nerves won't be affected. This ❑ highlights the importance of not only maintaining good blood glucose control but also other factors such as blood pressure, cholesterol and ❑ not smoking.

Healthy nerve Vs neuropathic nerve

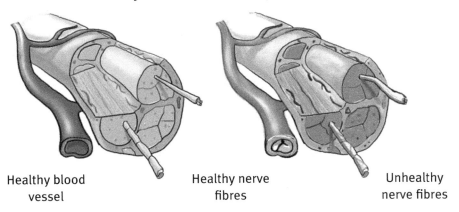

Healthy blood vessel   Healthy nerve fibres   Unhealthy nerve fibres

Our nervous supply to our feet comprises sensory, motor and autonomic nerves, all of which can be affected by diabetes.

Thus we can lose any combination – and ultimately all – of the following:

1. Sensory nerves:

   a. Light touch.
   b. Pain.
   c. Temperature differentiation.

2. Motor nerves (control of muscle action). There are 19 muscles in each foot. ❏

3. Autonomic nerves:
   a. Sweat glands.
   b. Proprioception, balance.

The nerves for each of these functions are different and are even dissimilar in structure so that they can be affected in diverse ways and at various times. This means therefore that it's possible for a person with diabetes to feel something lightly touching their foot like a feather and yet be oblivious to a sharp object sticking into their foot. ❏

It is vital that you, as a person with diabetes, are made aware of where ❏ you stand in the spectrum of neuropathy so you can risk assess your

life and take appropriate preventive measures to avoid problems. ❑
These preventive measures could be as simple as making sure you
don't walk around the house barefoot or even just being careful with
new shoes.

What are the dangers of diabetic neuropathy?

Loss of sensation is what comes to mind for most people when they
think of neuropathy and it is certainly a very important aspect. ❑
However neuropathy can also present in the following ways:

1. **Hypersensitivity.** You may experience a constant burning
   sensation often in a sock distribution on both feet. Sometimes ❑
   as the nerves become affected, there is a period of acute painful
   neuropathy which can present as hypersensitivity. This can be
   most uncomfortable and a patient may complain of anything from
   burning to stabbing pains to 'feeling like there are ants crawling all
   over my feet', to restlessness, muscle aches and sleeplessness due to ❑
   discomfort from contact with the bedclothes. Little can be done
   to relieve this although prescription creams such as Capsaicin can ❑
   help in some cases, as can cool footbaths. Bed cradles can also help
   by keeping the bedclothes off sensitive feet. Some medications can ❑
   also help so your consultant may be able to prescribe something
   that gives a little relief.

2. **Loss of sensation to pressure and pain – gentle or light touch
   and sharp touch.** As neuropathy worsens there is a gradual loss of
   sensation so that a person can be unaware of something touching ❑
   their feet or eventually something penetrating their feet. The hands
   can also be affected but the feet, as they are furthest away from
   the heart, will generally have the poorest circulation and therefore
   their nerves get affected first and worst. ❑

   You may think that sensation gives protection only against such
   things as stepping on something sharp and to a point (pun
   intended) that is correct. However a neuropathic foot will not
   warn the patient of other things such as the rubbing of a new shoe
   or a shoe that is slightly too short or indeed that bit of hard skin ❑

that has never really bothered you but has been getting worse and which in a normal foot would have started to give discomfort. Neuropathy can mask a problem so much that it is not unheard of for a diabetic to have investigatory x-rays for one thing only to be told that they are walking around on broken toe bones. ❏

3. **Loss of sensation to temperature.** The nerves that sense temperature can be affected and so extremes of temperature can ❏ go unnoticed in a person with diabetes. Something as simple as a hot water bottle in bed, a hot bath or even being too close to a fire ❏ can lead to very nasty burns and serious complications. Likewise a person may not be aware of just how cold their feet are getting and it is not uncommon in winter for the toes to become chilled to the point that bits of skin start to die and go cyanosed (blue) or even ❏ black. There is then a much greater risk of infection getting a hold in these areas of broken skin. ❏

4. **Loss of autonomic nerve function.** Along with chemicals in the blood, the autonomic nervous system plays a part in telling the brain when something is wrong so that the body has an early warning system and the central nervous system can orchestrate the right response at the correct time. ❏

The autonomic nervous system acts as a behind-the-scenes control system of involuntary functions such as digestion, heart rate, respiratory rate, and in the case of the feet, perspiration. ❏

So as neuropathy affects the autonomic nerves responsible for controlling the sweat glands as the disease progresses it is common for the person to sweat less and develop very dry skin. If they are already prone to hard skin this is likely to worsen and, as hard ❏ dry skin loses its natural suppleness, it is prone to cracking, which creates areas that are more likely to become infected and lead to more serious problems.

The autonomic nerves are also responsible for controlling a mechanism called the arterio-venous shunt which if not functioning properly will lead to the veins appearing very dilated and proud especially on the top of the foot. ❏

In affect, this means that in a neuropathic foot, the blood sometimes can be shunted directly from the arteries into the vein. If this is the case, then the blood is bypassing the capillaries and tissues it is supposed to be supplying with oxygen and nutrients meaning the superficial peripheral tissues are even more at risk of tissue death.

5. The motor nerves. These are the nerves that tell your muscles to work. In your body different muscle groups work against and in association with one another and in doing so they stabilise the joints. If some of the nerves are affected those muscles will not be told to work hard enough; they'll weaken and the joint they are supposed to stabilise becomes less stable. It's a bit like tug of war: normally the two teams are of equal strength, but if you tell one member on one side to stop pulling the other team will start winning. This effect in the feet leads to the muscles outside the feet pulling harder and classically leads to changes in foot shape. The common changes are toes starting to claw back and arches heightening, leading to deformity and subsequent areas of high pressure. These changes can cause greater risk of the damage that can come from increased pressure.

So what's the big problem?

Neuropathy can present with changes in any of these areas and each has its own issues which have worse risks associated than in a similar person who is not diabetic.

I have devised a seven-point home check system (see Chapter 15) which should help reduce the rate of deterioration of your foot health and help you to act on the awareness you are getting from reading this book. Alternatively visit **www.undefeeted.org/videos** and watch the tutorials on how to perform the tests. Of the seven tests two pertain to checking for loss of sensory function. I will also include a third test because of its importance although there is no protocol for carrying it out safely at present.

1) **The 'touch the toes' test as promoted by Diabetes UK.** Credit should be given to Dr Gerry Rayman and his team at Ipswich Hospital whose research showed that a simple test involving touching a person's toes very lightly while they have their eyes closed is a reliable way of

indicating if there is loss of sensory protection. For details of this test see Chapter 14 or visit **www.undefeeted.org/selftests**.

2) **Temperature sensation.** Again with your eyes shut your friend touches your feet alternately with a cold object such as a metal ❏ spoon and then with a plastic pen or similar. Before touching the feet, get the patient to feel the difference in their wrist. You should be able to tell the difference in temperature. If you can't this is cause for concern in a person with diabetes.

3) **Sharp/blunt discrimination.** This test is usually done by a podiatrist using a neurotip. It involves touching the feet randomly with either a sharp object or a blunt one. The person says whether they can feel it and whether it feels sharp or blunt. Although a person may pass ❏ the touch the toes test sometimes they are unable to feel sharp touch.

Some may say that a home test for this would be a valuable addition to a person's self-testing regime. At present there are no instruments available to test this safely in a non-clinical setting. Suggestions have been made such as cutting a cocktail stick in half and touching the feet in various places with extreme caution.

However I cannot endorse that as it would be possible to puncture the delicate skin of a person with neuropathy and peripheral vascular disease. It's unlikely, but it is better to err on the side of caution. As we will read in the next chapter, if the skin was broken infection could then flood in. So for that reason I would dissuade you from self-testing for sharp sensation.

I hope that someone will develop a safe means of carrying out this important test at home. In the meantime you would be wise to let your podiatrist do it annually.

Another useful test involves testing the autonomic nervous system with the use of a special chemical pad called a neuropad which changes colour in the presence of sweat. As the sweat glands are controlled by the autonomic nerves, it follows that if the skin is especially dry as in the case of autonomic nerve dysfunction, then the pad won't be activated to change colour thus giving an indication of that dysfunction.

The majority of diabetics I encounter have a vague awareness that they may lose sensation in their feet but have never been told how this may present and what to do to minimise the effects.

Firstly I have to assume that you are as active as possible and are doing your utmost to control your blood glucose levels as that is the best way of preventing nerve damage. The problem is that many people have diabetes for a number of years before they are diagnosed. During that time they won't necessarily be eating correctly with the consequence that long-term high blood sugars are likely to have caused some nerve damage even before they are diagnosed. Indeed at Circle Podiatry we insist on initial and then subsequent annual sensory and vascular tests and regularly pick up on someone who has lost sensation. A referral to their GP often reveals that person is diabetic without knowing it.

Jericho foot

There's a rare and devastating condition that I want to warn you about because it can affect anyone who has developed neuropathy. Its effects can be minimised if the right action is taken early enough. This is the development of a Charcot joint or osteoarthropathy. To help explain it I like to call it Jericho foot.

In the Bible there's an account of the destruction of Jericho, a fortified city, by the Israelites. Jericho had big stone walls so the people inside felt safe and the Israelites must have wondered if they'd be able to conquer it. Likewise most of us walk around on good strong feet that have done their job all our lives and we don't have any reason to worry about them holding out until we are very old.

The Israelites camped outside the town and the people inside felt secure. Then comes the game changer – God intervenes and tells the Israelites to march around the city every day for six days. This they did and nothing seemed to happen. You can imagine the people inside jeering at them. In Jericho foot an initial injury such as a trip or knock can be enough to start a hidden response and because of your neuropathy you're not really aware of anything happening – yet unbeknown to you your foot is about to collapse.

Likewise on the seventh day the people of Jericho would have felt comfortable expecting the same outcome as the previous six days. But on this day God had told the Israelites that they should march around the city seven times shouting and blowing trumpets. As they did that the walls came tumbling down and the city was destroyed. Likewise when a person develops a Jericho foot the joints disintegrate, the ligaments give way and the bones collapse leaving the foot a bit like the piles of rubble that would once have been the walls of Jericho. Even more frightening in a person developing a Jericho joint, they may not need to wait for seven days after the initial injury for this devastation to occur.

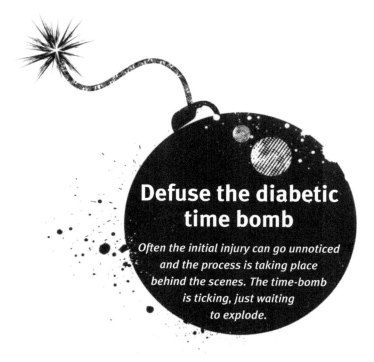

Defuse the diabetic time bomb

Often the initial injury can go unnoticed and the process is taking place behind the scenes. The time-bomb is ticking, just waiting to explode.

Don't laugh like my friends did but recently I fell down the stairs, which is a bit embarrassing at my age. My personal trainer had put me through it a couple of days previously and I woke up really stiff and sore. I slipped on my way down the stairs and my left foot saved me by jamming up against the staircase spindle. I don't have neuropathy, although my latest check suggests some early background changes, but I was well aware that an injury like that could so easily lead to a Jericho foot. I did what I would recommend any person with diabetes to do and got it checked out using an infrared thermometer. All was well but had it not been the case I would have been off to hospital to get an x-ray and bone scan to see what was damaged.

A colleague recently recounted the story of a nineteen-year-old girl who tripped, didn't get the care or tests done needed for a correct diagnosis and went on to develop a Jericho foot. Shortly afterwards this young lady had to have an amputation of her lower leg.

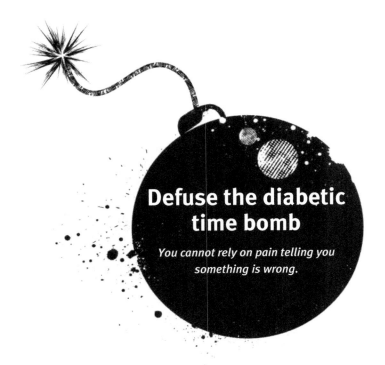

Defuse the diabetic time bomb

You cannot rely on pain telling you something is wrong.

The three stages of Jericho foot.

There are three stages to the condition which can affect any of the following joints: the ankle, hind foot, mid-foot, forefoot, toes and also the knee.

Acute stage. The problem area will usually be gradually affected but the changes can happen quickly too. It will appear red, hot and swollen with or without pain depending on the neuropathy. The temperature of the ❏ affected joint will usually be at least two degrees Celsius higher than the ❏ surrounding area. During this phase there is a lot of bony destruction taking place and it is of paramount importance that the patient is seen immediately as the foot needs to be supported using a cast. This will prevent ❏ the bones and ligaments from collapsing. They are already deteriorating and if the situation is not taken care of the joints could collapse later on, leaving the person with even worse deformity, instability and fractures. ❏

A successful outcome from a Charcot attack relies on the following things happening:

- A diagnosis as early as possible. ❏
- Early intervention. ❏
- Prevention of deformity. ❏
- Accommodating any deformities that did occur. ❏
- Possible correction of any deformity. ❏

A succeful resolution relies on an early diagnosis which in turn is more likely if you are already in the sweet spot, realising you are at risk of a Charcot, knowing what it is and what to do and that prompt ❏ action is critical.

So you need to know if you have neuropathy and are at more risk of it occurring. Then you need to know what to look for. A Charcot joint will usually be triggered by a traumatic event such as a knock, trip, or even just ❏ increased activity, for example following a period in hospital or perhaps a sudden increase in exercise as part of your weight loss programme.

Alarm bells should be ringing if the foot becomes red, swollen and hot. Often people don't worry about these symptoms and, because they may have no pain, don't seek help until the joint is irreversibly ❏ destroyed and the foot changes shape. They then get worried and trot – or rather limp – along to their doctor after the damage has been done

It is better to be safe than sorry and if you suspect a Charcot is possible then, as a matter of urgency, go to your diabetic clinic or accident and ❏ emergency department. If you have profound neuropathy then insist ❏ on an x-ray but stress you are a diabetic with neuropathy as in the early stages the x-ray may appear normal. A bone scan will tell the doctor more but is not very specific so ideally insist on an MRI which will show exactly what is going on and where. ❏

As soon as you suspect a Charcot then you must rest and certainly not bear any weight on that foot. If necessary use crutches or an upturned broom to support yourself. Continued weight bearing activity could ❏ cause further fractures, dislocations and ultimately severe deformity ❏ which can be prone to ulceration.

If caught in the early acute stage then the foot will be placed in a cast. Casting the foot does not reduce the reaction but does mean that at ❏ the end of the active phase the foot should reset in a more normal position. The earlier this is done the better so early diagnosis is critical and day one is better than day five.

Resolution phase.

On average during the resolution phase the cast stays on for three months or until there is only one degree temperature difference between the affected and good limbs.

Once the cast has come off the patient has to be encouraged to rest and only start walking with caution. It can take up to six months to calm down and resolve. Here patience is definitely a virtue. Friends and family should discourage you from doing too much.

Jericho / Charcot foot

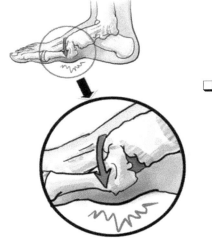

Sharp jagged bits of bone protrude from inside the foot causing recurrent trauma within the foot. Ulceration is also known to be quite common.

Rehabilitation stage.

Often at the end of an episode of Charcot osteoarthropathy a person is left with a deformed foot which is now even more prone to pressure points and subsequent danger areas for callus formation and ulceration. The most common is the rocker bottom foot as in the diagram. The bone surfaces often develop sharp protuberances which then press from within the foot on the soft tissues overlying them causing ulceration and necrosis which can be very dangerous.

The person should carry on with the process of rehabilitation. The podiatrist will try to offload these new areas of high pressure using pads stuck to the foot or accommodative orthotics to reduce the chance of the wound reopening.

A good lookout should be kept on the unaffected leg as it will naturally be favoured and can become traumatised itself forming an ulcer or even another Charcot joint.

Occasionally surgery may be undertaken after careful consideration to remove any sharp bony growths or even to fix the bones together, but surgery has its risks and is only undertaken after careful consideration ❏ as a final option.

Neuropathy is the big game changer in your walk with diabetes. Try to manage your diabetes to avoid it setting in but if you have already lost sensation then take to heart all the advice and put in place ways ❏ of protecting yourself. These will be discussed in Part Three.

Neuropathy changes everything: from not being aware of a trauma, to not having any tenderness or fever in an infection, not sensing gangrene or a heart attack, or the effects of hypoglycaemia.

If trauma and subsequent internal malfunctions are not sensed then diagnosis and treatment will be delayed. You and your diabetic foot care team have then missed the window of opportunity in which to prevent further tissue death.

Exercise: get into the sweet spot.

Go through the tick boxes in this chapter and answer the questions or complete the statements below.

1. What is the most important thing that you have learned in this chapter?

....

....

....

....

2. Which main risk factor have you become aware of?

....

....

....

....

3. The one big thing I am going to start/stop doing is

....

....

....

....

If you need to break that down into several steps, please go ahead and note them below. Make sure to add the date by which you intend to achieve each of those steps.

....

....

....

....

Chapter 11:
Infection.

A foot infection is a nightmare for a person with diabetes. The complications associated with infection in the foot and lower limb are truly a time-bomb just waiting to explode into a host of fearful consequences. The other complications we have explored can all predispose the person to subsequent infection. Once infected a person with diabetes, because they are immune suppressed, will not be able to fight infection and so it will spread not only over a bigger surface area but also to deeper places that are hidden from view. Not only do people with diabetes become more susceptible to infection, they often don't realise there is a problem as they can't feel it and maybe can't see it, thus allowing it to really get a foothold.

Just as attackers can penetrate a fort's defences through its weak spots, bacteria and microorganisms find it much easier to invade the tissues of the diabetic foot. Our skin is our first line of defence and normally does a wonderful job of keeping infections out and healing, but, as discussed previously, changes caused by diabetes can mean a break down in the skin's protective structure and a reduced healing rate once that breakdown has occurred.

Indeed an infection can often be the reason why people get tested and diagnosed in the first place.

These are some classic portals of entry for an infection:

1. Skin too wet. If the feet sweat too much, the space between the toes can become macerated or soggy. In extreme cases of hyperhidrosis (excess sweating) the soles of the feet can become white as the skin there becomes macerated.

Wherever possible shower before bed so you are not putting damp feet into your shoes. If you must take a shower before putting shoes ❏ on make sure you dry your feet well, especially between the toes. ❏ And be careful! It's easy to damage the delicate skin even with a towel. I tell my patients to use a piece of folded kitchen paper to ❏ dry between their toes as it absorbs well and will tear before your ❏ skin does. See Chapter 14 for more tips on what to do if you suffer from sweaty feet or sogginess between your toes.

2. **Dry skin.** Neuropathy associated with diabetes (see Chapter 10) can make the skin too dry, which can lead to cracks that can let bacteria in. If you are prone to hard or dry skin then start to apply ❏ a suitable foot cream with a high urea content every day. Initially apply once a day rubbing it in well and avoiding getting any ❏ between your toes. If it doesn't improve sufficiently, apply it twice daily. If you're not sure it is helping then just do one foot and note the difference after a couple of weeks. ❏

3. **Wound from a knock or stubbing the toes**. Wearing slippers around the house not only stops sharp objects penetrating the skin ❏ but also those horrible times when you catch your little toe on a piece of furniture. Another tip here is not to have too cluttered a house; a thorough clear out is always a good idea. Think about where you tend to leave things out and train your spouse, kids and ❏ pets not to leave things lying around.

4. **Ingrowing nails.** A toe nail can either curl in to form an involuted shape or have a sharp corner left from poor nail cutting. Both of ❏ these scenarios can lead to a break in the skin and subsequently a ❏ wound that is open to infection.

5. **Athletes foot.** A fungal infection that is not dangerous in itself but, as the skin can break, it is easy for a secondary bacterial infection ❏ to enter.

6. **Burns** including sunburn can blister and form an open wound. ❏

7. **Blisters** caused by new activities, new shoes or a foot that is functioning abnormally because of a bad structure. ❏

8. **Areas of high pressure/callus formation.** Areas of high pressue ❑ can cause a wound fairly quickly. For example, a shoe putting pressue on the foot or an extended period of being bed or chair bound causing pressure sores. High pressure over time can cause hard skin to build up which thickens thus increasing pressure even more leading to increased pressure on the deeper tissues and ultimately a breakdown (death) of those tissues.

9. **Thickened toenails** can be caused by one-off traumatic events, gradual repetitive trauma over a number of years and fungal ❑ infection. Once thick they are likely to have pressure on them from footwear and can ulcerate under the nail, which leads to infection. ❑

10. **Puncture wounds.** As the foreign body enters your flesh it can ❑ easily carry bacteria in with it and even when it is removed it leaves behind a little culture of bugs deep in your tissues which can then secretly multiply and spread the infection even into the bone (see ❑ page 154).

11. **Verrucae,** although not that dangerous in themselves, can cause problems as most treatments for them involve trying to kill off ❑ the skin cells that are hosting the virus. In effect we are trying to create a wound, which may not heal well in a person with diabetes. This is why nearly all over-the-counter treatments for verrucae will have a warning that tells people with diabetes not ❑ to use them.

12. **Blood-borne infection**. The foot infection can cause further ❑ infection elsewhere in the body or an infection elsewhere can spread to the foot

13. **Self inflicted** – often from DIY treatments, picking at nails or ❑ callus, or cutting nails too short.

Whatever the mode of invasion by the infection, it is of vital importance that it is tackled quickly otherwise in a person with ❑ diabetes it is likely to colonise and spread rapidly to other deeper tissues with serious consequences. A matter of 24-hours in seeking ❑ help can be the difference between an infection clearing up and the ❑ loss of the limb. The problem often is that the person doesn't seek help early enough as they don't feel any pain and so don't perceive they have a problem. They haven't taken on board the risk they face.

I just had a call from a friend whose husband is away on business in another country. He has type 2 diabetes and has told his wife that he's had a nasty insect bite on his leg. This occurred three days before and even though it was causing considerable pain, he still hadn't done anything. My friend sent me some photos of the sting which was red, angry and weeping, far more so than you would expect from a simple insect bite. I told her that because of her husband's diabetes it needed to be dealt with fast as it could deteriorate quickly to the point of needing serious surgery, hospitalisation or even amputation. I shared the idea of an iceberg infection where, just like a real iceberg has only ❏ a small part visible above the water, so too you can only see a small proportion of the problem, the rest is under the skin in the deeper ❏ tissues, possibly running rampant in the sugar-rich environment.

On further discussion her husband told her that he was feeling feverish and unwell. So the infection was bad enough to affect his ❏ whole body. I told her that he needed antibiotics straightaway and had to get to a hospital urgently.

Shortly afterwards I got the call to say that he was being stubborn and wouldn't go until after work the next day. If you as a person with diabetes ever get into a situation like that and refuse to take action, ❏ you are lighting the fuse of the time-bomb.

What would you do if you had two choices of how to cross a field full of landmines? Would you cut straight across because you wanted to get there quickly? Or would you take the more difficult path around the edge, which is harder and will take longer, but ensures your safe arrival at the other side?

Only time will tell how my friend's husband fairs, he or you may be lucky this time: but why play Russian roulette with your future? Just stop to think about what life would be like with only one leg. Go ahead: wiggle your toes around inside your shoes. Look back at your lifeline exercise in Part One and then look ahead... How would your life change if you lost a foot?

Why diabetics must take small infections seriously:

1. Have you ever wondered what happens to swabs and specimens taken by doctors and other health professionals? Apart from looking for the microorganism the laboratory will try to grow the bug so they can identify it and know what will best kill it. To do this they prepare little dishes of agar which is a nutrient and sugar-rich jelly-like substance (i.e. they make a perfect environment for the bugs to grow and multiply). In the same way **the wound of a diabetic provides an ideal sugar-rich environment on which the bacteria can thrive.** ❏

2. If you have peripheral vascular disease, your **ischemia** (poor blood supply) will mean the white blood cells that fight infection can't reach the site as easily. ❏

3. If you have any **neuropathy** you won't feel the need to rest the foot and so are likely to continue using it causing more damage and the infection to spread. ❏

4. The infection is often contained in quite tight compartments in the foot and the build up of pressure from any inflammation and pus formation will put pressure on the blood vessels, causing further ischemia. ❏

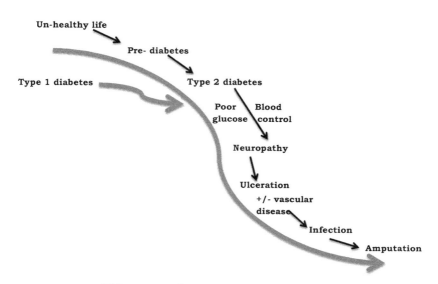

Slippery slope to amputation.

Once the diabetic foot has been wounded it's on a slippery slope. And for someone with neuropathy the wound may not have happened at all if they'd been able to feel any pain. The wound fails to heal and so provides a portal of entry for bacteria to cause a localised infection which then spreads and can become severe enough to threaten the person with loss of limb or even life.

When the infection is at the local stage, treatment could be some debridement (cutting away any dead tissue and removing any foreign bodies; e.g. glass, thorns, splinters) coupled with oral antibiotics.

As the infection spreads stronger injectable antibiotics will often be required with the wound being checked and redressed more regularly.

If the infection becomes severe then you would be hospitalised on intravenous antibiotics, often requiring surgical debridement of any necrotic (dead) tissue. The wound would need regular monitoring. It is usual at this stage for the wound to look much worse. Previously you could only see the tip of the iceberg yet all the necrotic tissue hidden beneath the skin has to be removed if the wound is going to have a chance to heal. So a small surface wound of a few millimetres may necessitate debridement in which it becomes an open wound 10-15 cm wide and 1-2 cm deep, where deeper tissues have been destroyed.

The one time I think it's best to be pessimistic is with wounds in people with diabetes. Always assume the worst case scenario: that you can only see one quarter of the wound, that it is infected with some horrible bug, that it is spreading, even that it may require amputation. Then do all you can to prevent that nightmare from becoming reality. I would prefer my clients to cry wolf and hassle me with minor problems rather than keeping quiet and turning up one day with a foot that cannot be saved.

Exercise: get into the sweet spot.

What I want you to do right now is revisit the tick boxes in this chapter and answer the questions or complete the statements below.

1. What is the most important thing that you have learned in this chapter?

....

....

....

....

2. Which main risk factor have you become aware of?

....

....

....

....

3. The one big thing I am going to start/stop doing is

....

....

....

....

If you need to break that down into several steps, please go ahead and note them below. Make sure to add the date by which you intend to achieve each of those steps.

....

....

....

....

Chapter 12:

Be on guard.

Please make sure to have a pen to hand and tick any box that is relevant to you in this section – I hope you're doing that anyway, but it's especially important for this chapter. Keep calm if you have to tick most of the boxes, in my experience many people do.

Hopefully you are now aware of all the risks and are forming good habits so you can manage them. By the way habits take time to form and this is especially true if you don't feel any real benefit from them as is the case with the diabetic foot; either there are no noticeable changes because it has a gradual effect or because the person literally ❏ can't feel anything because of neuropathy. It's not easy – but it can be done.

Even with the best ever habits and attention to our feet in our daily routines there are some factors that can put even the most diligent person at risk. I have named this chapter 'Be On Guard' as some events can't be predicted but their outcome will largely be dictated by your awareness and subsequent action. ❏

A classic example happened to me the other day when I was putting new rollers on a curved glass shower door. Stupidly I was doing it wearing just a pair of shorts. The first door went on fine but as I turned the second one upside down it shattered into thousands of pieces which went everywhere including over me. Little shards of glass stuck in my arms and back and my bare feet were surrounded and covered by glass. I couldn't move because if I did I would be standing on it. Luckily my wife was upstairs so I got her to throw me a pair of old shoes. I lifted one foot and carefully brushed it off with a towel. When we were sure there was no glass left on it I put it in the shoe and repeated the same process for the second foot. Amazingly

I got no cuts on my feet but I imagined what would have happened had I been alone and forced to move barefoot. My challenge and yours is to risk assess in future and wear shoes (or get someone else to do it for me – my wife's suggestion!) ❏

One other point I should make is that after we had cleared up I had to assess if the shoes were worth keeping. They weren't as the glass had penetrated deep into the soles. So they were binned. ❏

So remember, it's important to wear slippers or shoes at all times and to ensure your family knows the importance of owning up and telling you if there has been a mishap. ❏

I recall one patient at a hospital outpatients department on the day after Boxing Day who had already had a previous partial amputation of one foot. He knew he couldn't feel anything but had helped clear up a glass his daughter had broken. He hadn't bothered putting on shoes and sure enough he'd trodden on a piece of glass which had ❏ cut the sole of his foot. He didn't feel it. The first he knew of it was when he saw the smears of blood on the kitchen floor. He said it had happened three days earlier on Christmas Eve but hadn't rung because he thought the department would be busy and he could look after it himself.

It is essential to address a wound early. His delay in going for treatment meant the small cut had become a gaping deep infected wound which ❏ needed intravenous antibiotics and surgical debridement of dead tissue necessitating admission to hospital and missing the rest of the festive period. At this point it could either heal up or need a further amputation. If a wound like this does heal it will leave a scar and an area vulnerable to further ulceration and infection.

As a person with diabetes you need to realise just how vulnerable you are and that should motivate you to risk assess certain scenarios you find yourself in. ❏

For most of us our daily routine doesn't change that much and once we have done the initial risk assessment and maybe changed some habits and environmental factors, we should be set up for as safe a life as possible living in the diabetic sweet spot. ❏

However it's at times of change when you are probably most at risk, when your environment may be unfamiliar, or you may be asking more of your feet than usual.

These can be broken down into the following categories:

Change of external macro environment – holidays and seasons. The change in a person's environment can put them at increased risk that they wouldn't be as vulnerable to in a more familiar environment. It's not top of most people's agenda but we would do well to carry out a simple risk assessment when we change our environment.

As a person with diabetes you need to work out what level of risk you are at and what action you need to take. Does this mean we wrap ourselves in cotton wool and never do anything risky? I think not; but my philosophy is that we become aware of the risks and then ask ourselves the following three questions:

a. What is the best outcome?

b. What is the worst outcome?

c. And what is the most likely outcome?

The worst outcome could be either very unlikely or very likely and this should help us decide whether it's worth taking the risk. So let's have a look at some of the risky situations we can find ourselves in regarding our feet and diabetes. The factors we have talked about in previous chapters, such as neuropathy, will exacerbate any risk.

Holidays.

1. Bashing your foot. As we all know our little toe can often get stubbed and in my experience people often do it when in an unfamiliar place. When on holiday we are in an environment that is new to us and are more likely to stub our toes. If you are diabetic a simple thing like this can lead to a wound that doesn't heal or even bring on a Charcot joint. You need to work out what you can do to minimise the risk. This may be ensuring you wear sturdy slippers or indoor shoes or having someone point out where furniture is if you are partially sighted.

2. Holiday feel-good factor. You're meant to be barefoot aren't you? ❏ It's a great temptation to go barefoot in a hot country or on a sandy beach. Obviously you risk treading on something sharp but what about if the tarmac gets too hot and you're not able to feel it? ❏ Amputations have happened because of this. It is far better to wear sandals or flip flops.

3. Swimming in the sea. It may pay to wear some waterproof sandals or wet shoes. You never know what other holiday makers have discarded and not all beaches are covered in golden sand but have sharp stones and pieces of shell, not to mention sea anemones whose spines can play havoc with a foot even if the person doesn't ❏ have diabetes.

4. Holiday footwear. Whether a beach holiday or not we may need to wear different shoes which may be new or at best ones we are not used to. This can lead to anything from blisters and pressure points to postural issues higher up the body. Perhaps we would be better ❏ wearing the shoes in a bit at home before the holiday. Children's ❏ walking boots may not fit as well as they did last year and even an adult's feet can change if the person's arches have dropped or the feet become swollen; so what fitted and was suitable last year isn't necessarily suitable this year and could cause a problem. ❏

5. Increased activity although good may be too much too quickly leading to injuries of either the feet or higher in the body. If you are going trekking and are not used to that level and type of walking it ❏ may be worth stepping up your mileage before you leave.

6. Decreased activity may lead to heightened blood sugar levels. ❏

7. And what about the temptation of **all that lovely food** especially if you're returning to somewhere you went before your diagnosis? A lot of the fun on holiday can be down to the delicious local cuisine. But if recently diagnosed, you were probably non diabetic the last time you ate at that fantastic restaurant and you will need to watch your food choices carefully. ❏

8. Chilling or sunburn. Have you ever been out in the sun unaware of how burnt you have become until you get in the shower and go to bed? Then you feel it! If you have neuropathy you may not feel it at all on your feet and so you stay in the sun too long the next day causing blistering which can lead to infection. ❏

9. **Insect or other bites** can also be serious and precautions should be taken to deter them from choosing you. If you do get bitten on the foot apply a cream like Anthisan which will lessen the itching. The bite itself will probably heal but often it's the scratching that introduces a secondary bacterial infection. ❏

10. **Picking up nasty infections**. You probably associate verrucae/plantar warts and athletes foot with swimming pools and changing rooms. These are contagious. Yes you need to be careful of changing rooms at gyms and pools but what about holiday homes and hotels? It may be wise to wear flip flops in these areas. ❏

1. Seasons

The seasons can cause more problems than you might expect with both direct and indirect factors. ❏

a. Summer:

a. Direct factors such as **sunburn** in the summer (perhaps not so much in the UK!) ❏

b. More likely to walk **barefoot** and risking puncture wounds. ❏

c. Less supportive shoes can lead to overloading of the foot as well as postural issues. ❏

d. A **change in the micro environment** can cause increased sweating which in turn creates the perfect environment for athletes foot. Athletes foot can easily cause breaks in the skin which can allow bacterial infection in. ❏

e. Hot weather will increase sweating and so predispose to athletes foot whereas **open back shoes can lead to drying** of the heels and callus build-up with risk of fissuring (cracking). ❏

f. This summer we had the opportunity to enjoy several barbeques and thanks to that I can add this advice. Once it fell to my lot to do the cooking. It wasn't long before I realised I was getting spat on by the sizzling meat with hot fat landing on the tops of my feet. I was glad I could feel it but some of you may not. ❏ Next time I risk assessed and got someone else to do it (thanks Johnny!) I could equally have chosen to put closed shoes on instead as protection. ❏

b. Winter:

a. **Chilling in the winter** is a common complication in a person if they have a degree of ischemia due to peripheral vascular disease where the blood can't get the nutrients and oxygen to the wound. ❏ Also areas of high pressure can be prone to chilling as the blood may be squeezed out of an area by overloading either under the foot or from a tight upper. ❏

b. **Chilblains**, although not as common in the UK as in the days prior to central heating, can still present and are usually a result of the feet getting too cold and then being warmed up too quickly. They can become very itchy and you should take care not to scratch and break the skin. ❏

c. **Changing shoe type** can lead to developing pressure points, blisters or callus. ❏

d. **Falling on ice** can cause Charcot joints or just immobilise a person for some time which in turn raises blood sugars. ❏

e. **Change of local micro environment**: holidays and seasons, new hosiery and shoes. ❏

2. Random acts of danger.

a. **Pets; Trojan horse syndrome**. You may be familiar with the story from *The Iliad* where, during the Trojan War, the Greeks built a huge hollow horse then cunningly sailed away – but only just out of view of Troy. Meanwhile Sinon was left behind and persuaded the Trojans that the horse was an offering to the goddess Athena and would make Troy impregnable. The Trojans accepted the gift and dragged it into the city. Unbeknown to them some of the best

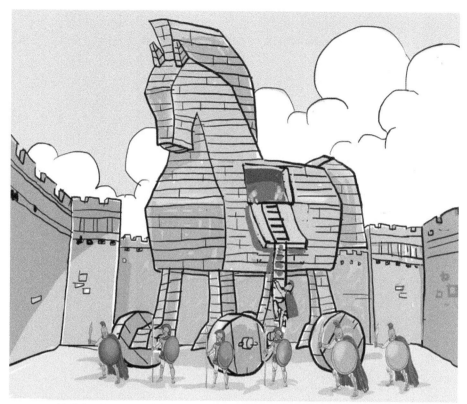

"Right lads you attack the muscle, you the tendon and I'll get the bone!"

Greek fighters had hidden inside the horse, they crept out in the dead of night and opened the gates, allowing their army, which had sailed back under the cover of darkness to enter the city and destroy it.

The gates of the diabetic foot can easily be left wide open to the army of bacteria in your sock and shoe by wounds such as standing on a sharp object that penetrates the skin. Whether it remains in or not it may well have deposited within your sugar-rich tissues some bacterial soldiers that start destroying your foot-fort from within creating an open gate for other bugs. Just like the Trojan horse which seemed inoffensive to the people of Troy so may a pet hair that has worked its way into your skin. Dog hairs and even human hairs can work their way into the skin and cause deep infection.

They usually present with either the end embedded in the skin or just a little sticking out, when pulled gently I have known up to one inch of hair to come out. Pets, particularly those with coarse hair, can be the cause of your amputation.

Coarse hairs can literally work their way into your skin.

Jean, a patient who comes in roughly every six months, is a well spoken and well dressed lady. Yet every visit without fail I debride (remove with a scalpel) her hard skin and find not one but two or three dog hairs embedded in her foot. I was perplexed as to ❑ why Jean suffered so frequently with this problem when other dog lovers didn't.

I took the foot bed out of her shoes to find half a dog's worth of hair within each one. I think I asked if her dog was bald now! ❑ I suspected that her slippers were the same and advised her to vacuum all her footwear thoroughly and make it a habit to do it once a month. Sure enough I rarely see her now and never with ❑ that problem. Animal lovers: add another household chore to your list and if your pet moults vacuum the inside of your shoes. ❑

Whilst on the subject of pets a particularly gross piece of advice is not to let your animal (dogs have a tendency) lick your feet and legs especially if you have an open wound. You don't know which part ❑ of their anatomy (actually you probably do...) they were licking before turning to your wound!

3. Yourself.

    i. Self-operating. Many a foot or leg has been lost by self-treatments gone wrong. If you are diabetic **don't self-operate** unless your podiatrist has actually advised you to. This is unlikely ❑ except for nail cutting and then only if you are not at increased risk. Additionally never use corn plasters or verruca treatments without professional advice - they are designed to burn your skin and easily cause a wound that can get infected and never heal.

ii. Nail cutting. Make sure you cut straight across using nail clippers (not scissors) and never go down the sides. Don't cut too short or conversely leave to grow too long. File any rough edges with an emery board/nail file. ❏

iii. Lack of good hygiene. Wash your feet (including between the toes) as part of your five-minute daily self-check routine (see page 195). ❏ Dry carefully between the toes using kitchen paper. If you find it ❏ difficult to reach to wash properly use an extra soft toothbrush gently between the toes. A kids' one will have the softest bristles and a smaller head. Do be careful not to rub too hard or damage ❏ the skin.

4. **Your career or job.** There are three aspects to this. Firstly you may be in a job where you are more susceptible to external trauma. Safety boots have helped prevent many amputations so don't be tempted to give them a miss. On the other hand I have seen ❏ instances where a too small boot has been worn and has caused a wound or is in the process of doing so by building up callus which ❏ can ulcerate. Some companies insist on you wearing the boots they ❏ issue. Insist that they fit and if not get your podiatrist or GP to write a letter asking that you choose and buy your own from a wider choice ensuring you get the correct fit. Jobs requiring a lot of kneeling can also lead to nail problems and callus build up on the toes, especially the big toes.

Conversely some of us have sedentary jobs and over time inactivity can lead to weight gain which itself can be a factor in the development and deterioration of your diabetes. Or you may find ❏ that a sudden increase in activity, say you start a new sport, can lead to such things as blisters and internal trauma such as plantar ❏ fasciitis or tendonitis.

Thirdly both ladies and gentlemen may be in a profession where they are expected to dress smartly and of course that includes the shoes. ❏ Men can usually get away with finding a suitable shoe but many ladies hobble around in shoes that are doing long-term damage as well ❏ as putting them at risk of problems such as ingrown nails; forefoot pain from overloading the metatarsal heads or the formation of a neuroma; blisters and changes to the bone or joints as in bunions, hammer and claw toes and heel bumps (see Chapter 14).

5. **Your lifestyle.** A sedentary lifestyle is not good for you. Also make sure you wear appropriate footwear for activities such as gardening ❑ and DIY. Do your own risk assessment before doing jobs at home ❑ or work that could potentially cause you harm.

6. **Your fashion.** High heels spring to most people's minds as a cause of problems later in life but also too pointed a shoe can cause ❑ issues as can too flat a shoe. Believe it or not sometimes we advise someone that a bit of a heel would be better for them (I am saying ❑ a bit – that is not a licence to go and buy skyscraper heels). Guys are not exempt either – their foot structure may mean that they will benefit from a bit of a heel too. Of course you need to be assessed to know what your foot type is and what would be best for you. Oh and by the way ladies I am not suggesting you can't ever ❑ wear high heels: just keep them for occasional use and be sensible with them. ❑

7. **Your family.** The bottom line is that you are responsible for you. ❑ If your family and friends love a doughnut every day it doesn't mean you have to have one. That said our families can be asked to be sensitive, and anyway eating more healthily will benefit them especially as they are at increased risk of developing diabetes as well. ❑

8. **Lack of routine podiatry care.** Many people put up with bits of hard skin and even corns. You as a person with diabetes may not ❑ feel them but it is critical that you get them treated regularly to ensure the build-up doesn't become too much and cause an ulcer. ❑ When you get a hard plaque of callus the skin is no longer supple (as it should be) and the forces of the shoe against it and even just the foot bending means the whole plaque moves which can lead to changes in the structure of the skin. I have seen blood blisters that ❑ have formed as a result of the shoe and hard skin pinching some healthy skin. Often all will be okay for some time and then a new

pair of shoes, or going on holiday will change the forces and cause a problem which could have been avoided.

❏

9. **Familiarity breeds contempt.** Many people put up with discomfort for years, for example paying minimal attention to areas of hard skin or cracks. It is easy for you to become so used to a problem that you don't realise that since your diagnosis it is now a threat and needs to be dealt with more conscientiously.

❏

What to do scenarios

Being prepared for any situation will usually determine whether or not the outcome is positive or negative. Below are some common scenarios that we hope not to find ourselves in and yet one day we just may do. So here are some useful tips of what to do if you experience a:

1. Wound.

You cause a wound on your foot or maybe just find one. The key action is to take action quickly. That action should include getting it seen by a podiatrist as soon as possible. Remember it may seem small to you but diabetic wounds can often be like icebergs with only the tip of the problem visible. Only a very small abrasion is enough to let in microscopic infections that can devastate the area. This can happen very quickly in someone with diabetes so get seen the same day if at all possible.

If you have only noticed the wound outside of normal working hours, either get it checked at your local A and E or bathe it in salt water (a strong solution of table salt will help draw out infection). Remove any obvious debris from the wound and check for any foreign bodies such as splinters, glass, china or grit. Make sure you get it seen professionally the next day, even if it disrupts your plans or means cancelling a holiday! It is better to get the all clear rather than letting something minor threaten your limb and livelihood and ability to go on holiday at all in the future.

If you are unsure about the cause, check your shoes both inside and out for loose things in the shoe and for sharp objects penetrating the sole.

2. Ulcer.

An ulcer could suddenly rear its ugly head due to a build up of pressure, for example, under a hard bit of callus or a thickened nail. People often put up with pain whilst the callus builds up or they have neuropathy and can't feel it and then one day become aware of a damp patch on their sock indicating that there is an ulcer deep beneath the hard skin or nail. As with all wounds, this is now a portal of entry for bacteria which if left alone can run riot hidden from view and infect deep into the foot. It is therefore critical that this is seen professionally as soon as possible. Sometimes the area can be temporarily offloaded using adhesive Chiropody felt with a hole cut in it over the wound to deflect the pressure away. Additionally, an antiseptic spray such as Savlon dry powder spray will help kill bacteria.

3. Verruca.

Verrucae are difficult to get rid of at the best of times and as most treatments rely on destroying the skin, the verruca is infecting, and a wound is often caused. This, of course, can be an issue in a person with diabetes who may not heal. For this reason, most over the counter treatments will warn you that they are not suitable for use on a diabetic foot. Don't be tempted to self treat. Get a professional opinion and guidance as to what can be done.

4. Ingrown Toe Nail.

This condition is normally very painful and so help is sought, but of course in the diabetic foot it may be pain free and allowed to get worse. There are different causes such as bad cutting of nails, picking at nails, and excessive curling across the width of a nail. All of these are in effect causing a piece of nail to dig into the flesh next to it. This can become a wound and is again prone to infection. As with the wounds above, bathing in strong salt solution will help prevent infection but most importantly get to see a podiatrist tomorrow or, better still, today. Often a simple procedure with no need for local anaesthetic can remove the offending piece of nail and everything heals up. Leaving the bit of nail sticking in doesn't allow the healing process to take place. Even in a person without diabetes, antibiotics alone are unlikely to resolve the issue and in the case of a person with diabetes, the infection can easily spread to the underlying bone.

5. Sogginess between the toes

Often toes can become tightly packed together either due to swelling, tight shoes or just the forces put on them whilst walking. This tightness means that the air is unable to help the areas between the toes dry out and the skin becomes damp and white looking. This is a perfect environment for both bacterial and fungal infections to thrive. Try to keep between the toes dry by not applying cream there and not having a shower just before putting shoes on. Leather soled shoes and cotton rich or woollen socks will help. You could try applying surgical spirit with a cotton bud if there is not an open wound.

6. Athlete's foot.

This can come on fairly quickly perhaps if our foot hygiene is not good enough or especially if our feet are too damp enclosed in shoes for too long or get neglected whilst we are away, or just because the floors we are treading on can be a source of infection. We may be in a hotter climate where our feet perspire more or maybe coming off the beach where bits of sand could have been left in between the toes which can irritate and cause small abrasions and allow the infection to get a grip. Over the counter creams and powders can help kill the fungus causing the infection.

7. Deformity.

The deformity itself generally does not cause as much alarm to the person as the problems associated with it such as pressure lesions. It is often then that the person notices that their foot is misshapen. Any changes should be checked out professionally.

This misshaping is unlikely to happen quickly except in the case of a Charcot jt forming (see Chapter 10). However, gradual changes in the shape of the feet can go unnoticed until one day you suddenly realise there is a problem often brought to your attention by a particular pair of shoes creating a wound from too much pressure or rubbing.

As with any wound, get it seen to quickly but also try to identify which shoe was the culprit and then however attached to them you are, bin them or at least take them to your podiatrist for their opinion. Sometimes you may be able to get away with getting them stretched over the area of the deformity.

Exercise: get into the sweet spot.

What I want you to do right now is revisit the tick boxes in this chapter and answer the questions or complete the statements below.

1. What is the most important thing that you have learned in this chapter?

....

....

....

....

2. Which main risk factor have you become aware of?

....

....

....

....

3. The one big thing I am going to start/stop doing is

....

....

....

....

If you need to break that down into several steps, please go ahead and note them below. Make sure to add the date by which you intend to achieve each of those steps.

....

....

....

....

Congratulations on getting this far!

Please revisit these summary pages once a year as you'll find different points stick in your mind or are more relevant at different points in your life. This book is not intended to end up under the short leg of a table: it is your foot care manual and will help you stay fit and healthy during your journey with diabetes. I don't even want to find it in a charity shop! It is yours and should be filled with notes that can help you create a healthy future even though you have diabetes.

Part Three:
Together Everyone Achieves More

Did you know that **50% of people with diabetes do not know they have it?** So it makes sense, whether you have diabetes or not, to commit to a proper health care plan.

If you do have diabetes then, with a sensible plan that's tailored to your needs (including daily maintenance, regular visits to a podiatrist, and your annual foot MOT), plus a little help from your friends, family and health professionals, you **can** stay safe and sound in the diabetic sweet spot. Read on to find out what you can do to help yourself, where you need to ask for assistance and when you need to **take action**.

It's the surest way to remain **Undefeeted™**.

Introduction:
Know where you stand.

By reading this book you are empowering yourself to beat the negative aspects of diabetes and are making sure you are prepared for whatever life may throw at you.

So far we have looked at what can go wrong in a general way but it is critical that you as an individual know exactly where you or your loved one stands because the advice will vary dependant on the effects to date ❏ in your body. As a person with diabetes and a podiatrist I share the view of the Society of Podiatrists and Chiropodists that every person with diabetes should have a thorough diabetic foot assessment every year. ❏

It's just like an MOT.[2] At the end of it we should be aware of any serious issues that need sorting out as well as receiving some sound professional advice.

The other day I sat in a queue of cars waiting for my MOT to be done. The guy in front was desperately trying to fit a bulb into the rear brake light knowing that the car would fail if it wasn't working. Often, if something isn't directly affecting us, we let it go. As a person ❏ with diabetes the biggest favour you can do yourself is become observant and break your habits of procrastination. ❏

If you don't have diabetes but someone in your family does then these checks are important for you too. If you have diabetes, regular check-ups of your feet are essential. Our cars have spare wheels or ❏ ways of preventing a flat tyre. Are you doing your best to prevent the equivalent of a flat tyre in your life? Medical science is still a long way from being able to offer you a foot transplant.

---

[2] For non-UK readers the MOT is an annual test done in the UK to ensure that any vehicle driven on the road is in a roadworthy condition. The test checks that the vehicle meets road safety and environmental standards and can only be performed by government approved MOT test centres.

I'll just read the book and do it myself.

You need more than a book. It is of paramount importance that **you**, Jane Doe or Jack the lad, have your unique feet checked professionally. No book can deal with all of your individual problems. This book was ❏ written with you in mind, but you can't beat a personal assessment by a fully qualified podiatrist. If your car suddenly developed a noise you may Google it, but the chances are you'll get it checked by a qualified mechanic because you don't want it to let you down. The more value you put on it the more urgently you will attend to it.

I know that annual check-ups at doctor's surgeries can be extremely scant – although they do vary remarkably. Systems such as the Traffic Light risk screening tool will be a great help in raising the standards of screening from differing professions in the future. Even so, **I CAN'T EMPHASIZE ENOUGH THE IMPORTANCE OF GETTING CHECKED OUT REGULARLY BY A PODIATRIST.** ❏

Chapter 13:
The foot MOT.

In the UK any car more than three years old has to have an MOT annually in order to be allowed on the road.

It is a thorough test and I'm sure it's led to better safety standards on our roads. It does however only check the car's roadworthiness at that exact moment; it's just a snapshot. The following day someone could cut a brake pipe and make the car unroadworthy. Likewise if you are told at your annual foot MOT that you are at low risk of developing problems it doesn't mean you can become blasé about your foot care or blood sugar control. Things can change quickly, especially for a ❏ person with diabetes.

Even the weather can have an effect. In the UK a foot which was deemed low risk in September when the ambient temperature was higher could, with only minor deterioration, become higher risk in ❏ December when it is considerably colder.

What to expect from a proper diabetic foot assessment.

When deciding to go and get your feet looked at it is worth asking what you will be checked for as some checks are more intensive than ❏ others. Some you may find extremely thorough while others may work below the standards set out in The Society of Chiropodists and Podiatrists guidelines (our professional body).

You may also be wondering who you should see – a chiropodist or a podiatrist? And what's the difference between them anyway?

Podiatrist or chiropodist – who should I see?

It's hardly surprising that people are confused as even within our profession there is some perplexity – if you ask five podiatrists and five chiropodists that question you'd probably get 10 different answers.

The general impression appears to be that a chiropodist deals with hard skin and nails whereas a podiatrist also addresses the gait and foot structure. Just to clarify here in the UK there is no difference between the two. The two names are interchangeable. In fact the Society of Chiropodists and ❏ Podiatrists voted on whether to drop 'chiropodist' from their name to help reduce public confusion. Apparently there were enough people within the profession favouring it to warrant keeping the two names.

Originally we were called chiropodists but podiatrist became more widely used to align us with the rest of the world such as the US and Australia. So there is no difference and you can see any chiropodist or podiatrist (registered in the UK with the Health and Care Professions Council or HCPC) who should provide a high level of care for your lower limbs.

In the UK there is no difference between chiropodists and podiatrists. The two names are interchangeable.

Prior to 2005 there was no protection of our title and there were two main routes to be able to practice, either a three-year degree (previously a diploma) or a five-week correspondence course. When the protection of title came in those who had only done the correspondence course were required to meet certain standards to ensure the protection of the general public. A large number did not meet this standard and so forfeited the right to call themselves either podiatrist or chiropodist. (It is illegal for them to do so or to suggest that they are able to provide chiropody/podiatry treatments.)

Many of these then chose to call themselves foot health practitioners. These ❏ practitioners are **not** regulated by the HCPC[3] and therefore in my opinion ❏ should be avoided.

---

[3] The HCPC is the UK-based body regulating the professions allied to medicine. It helps protect you and ensure you are treated appropriately, for example with properly sterilised instruments. You can find them at www.hpc-uk.org.

So now you know you should always see a podiatrist/chiropodist. One further point to note for UK readers is that our regulatory body has an accreditation scheme which some practices have attained. This means that those practices are working to the highest possible standards above and beyond the Society's minimum guidelines. You can find your nearest accredited practice at **www.scpod.org**. ❑

The Traffic Light System.

When you're deciding which podiatrist (or chiropodist) to book in with, it would be worth asking them if they're aware of the **Traffic Light System**. My friend and colleague Duncan Stang (National Diabetes Foot Coordinator for Scotland) introduced this risk stratification and triage system in Scotland. It's been very successful and has been taken up by many foot health professionals. It has been recognised by NICE (National Institute for Health and Care Excellence) and Diabetes UK and has been adopted throughout the rest of the UK. Following the screening process, the system ensures each patient is assigned a risk category according to their risk of developing a foot ulcer. Although not a full assessment Duncan's research shows that the tests within the Traffic Light System give sufficient information to allow the person to be screened, given a risk category and hence advice on how to ❑ best manage themselves. It also implements a treatment/management plan according to the patient's needs.

An online educational tool has been developed by **www.diabetesframe.org** to ensure that whoever is carrying out the screening is doing so in a standardised and evidence-based manner. This is important especially as sometimes the screening is carried out by someone who isn't a foot specialist or where time constraints mean the tests have to be prioritised.

I'll summarise this internationally recognised system for the minimal levels of tests that a person with diabetes should undergo once a year. The tests allow a health professional with minimal training to screen you for your risk status which will be communicated to you so you are aware of how at risk you are and what level of input from podiatry services you should be receiving. This is important if you want to live in the sweet spot and hopefully not develop any foot problems. It also allows you to be referred for further in-depth assessment or care as appropriate for your level of risk.

The Traffic Light System: know your risk rating.

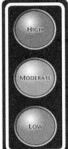

Your annual foot screening should tell you what level of risk you have been placed in. ❏

There are four levels of risk: ❏

- Low (green).
- Moderate or increased (amber).
- High (red).
- Active (the speed camera).

The screening looks at: ❏

1. Can you feel a 10g monofilament or vibration sensation?
2. Can the health professional palpate the pulses in your feet?
3. Has the foot any deformity?
4. Is there any significant callus?
5. Are there any signs of ulceration?
6. Is there any previous history of ulceration?
7. Do you feel any pain?
8. An inspection of your shoes.
9. Are you able to do your own self-care (i.e. can you reach and/or see your feet) or do you have someone who can help you?

After the assessment, you will be assigned to a risk level and an appropriate treatment/ management plan is put in place.

1. Green: low risk of developing active foot disease.

Definition: If you have no risk factors present then you are at low risk of any immediate active foot disease. On the traffic light diagram ❑ you would be green (bottom circle).

Action: You should have an annual screening by a suitably trained healthcare professional and have an agreed self management plan. You should also be provided with written and verbal education ❑ with emergency contact numbers and have appropriate access to a podiatrist if needed. ❑

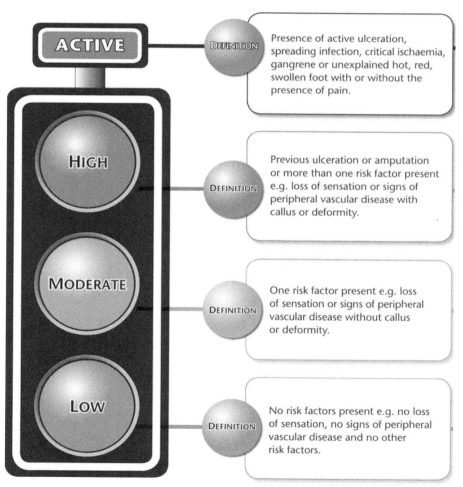

ACTIVE

DEFINITION — Presence of active ulceration, spreading infection, critical ischaemia, gangrene or unexplained hot, red, swollen foot with or without the presence of pain.

HIGH

DEFINITION — Previous ulceration or amputation or more than one risk factor present e.g. loss of sensation or signs of peripheral vascular disease with callus or deformity.

MODERATE

DEFINITION — One risk factor present e.g. loss of sensation or signs of peripheral vascular disease without callus or deformity.

LOW

DEFINITION — No risk factors present e.g. no loss of sensation, no signs of peripheral vascular disease and no other risk factors.

Produced by the Scottish Diabetes Group - Foot Action Group

2. Amber: moderate/increased risk of developing active foot disease.

Definition: If you have only one risk factor present then you are at moderate (increased) risk of developing any immediate active foot disease. You would be amber (middle circle) on the traffic light diagram. ❏

Action: Annual or 3-6 monthly assessment together with an agreed and tailored management/treatment plan (dependant on need) by a podiatrist or member of the foot protection team (FPT). You should ❏ also be provided with written and verbal education with emergency contact numbers. Referral should be made as necessary for specialist intervention.

3. Red: high risk of developing active foot disease.

Definition: If however you have more than one risk factor present and/or have previously had a foot ulcer or amputation then you are ❏ at high risk of developing immediate active foot disease. You would be the red light in the diagram (top circle).

Action: Annual or 1-3 monthly assessment together with an agreed and tailored management/treatment plan (dependant on need) by ❏ a podiatrist or member of the FPT. You should also be provided with written and verbal education with emergency contact numbers. Referral should be made as necessary for specialist intervention.

4. Speed camera: presence of active foot disease.

Definition: If you have active foot disease you will have any one of the following: ❏

a. Active ulceration.

b. Critical ischemia.

c. Gangrene.

d. Unexplained hot, red, swollen foot with or without pain.

e. Painful peripheral neuropathy.

f. Acute Charcot foot.

Action: Rapid referral to and management by a member of a multidisciplinary foot team. Have an agreed and tailored management/ ❏ treatment plan according to your needs. You should also be provided with written and verbal education with emergency contact numbers. Referral should be made as necessary for specialist intervention.

****

At the end of the screening you should be informed of your risk and what you can do. If you take action then you should be able to find your way back into the sweet spot.

> *"It's insanity to carry on doing the same thing and expect different results."*
>
> Albert Einstein.

Once a person's risk category changes so too should their self-care and their professional care plan should adjust to account for their ❏ new needs.

The screening above is excellent for tackling the huge numbers of people putting a strain on the NHS. However, a more detailed assessment will pick up problems earlier and you have a better chance of being safe from an early stage.

In my practice, Circle Podiatry, we use our gold standard to test everyone on their first visit irrespective of whether they have diabetes. This has the added benefit that sometimes we identify issues which can lead to a diagnosis of diabetes or another ailment long before the person would have been aware of it. In our hectic lives we will put up ❏ with tiredness for a long time before suspecting anything is wrong, yet it can be an indicator of diabetes.

Just today I saw a new patient for the first time, a gentleman in his late 60s who was concerned about a strange feeling on both sides of his forefoot. An initial look at his feet revealed a good general appearance with hairs on his big toes (indicating a healthy blood supply). The general condition of his skin was good.

However on closer inspection I found not one but two small cuts on the sole of his foot. He was not aware of any real discomfort there and on further investigation I located and removed two pieces of glass. I tested these areas using a monofilament (light touch test) which he could detect and yet when using a neuropen to test sharp touch he was unable to feel it.

Neuropathy can present in various ways and his initial complaint of feeling like he had a sock rolled up under his foot could be a sign of diabetic neuropathy. I questioned him further and found that he was also feeling incredibly tired and thirsty. I had already decided to refer him for diabetes tests and this extra information confirmed the need for me to do so.

I await his results and in the meantime it is wise for him and me to treat his wounds as if he has diabetes, just to be on the safe side. He left the clinic that day shocked but extremely grateful. He was prepared to face the facts so he could deal with his situation appropriately.

The majority of people who see me have no idea what to expect from an assessment and usually leave amazed at how complex and important the feet are. Let me share the experience with you as if you've come to my clinic today.

Gold standard tests.

Our receptionists welcome you and help you feel at ease while you fill out a form detailing your medical history. The practitioner greets you and shows you into the consulting room. So far it's probably not too dissimilar to your experience of the dentist. If it's your first visit to a podiatrist you may be feeling nervous or even scared and clients regularly say they feel ashamed of their feet. There's no need for that as most of our work does not involve any discomfort and with 27 years' experience I have pretty much seen it all.

Now you are in the consulting room you'll be asked to remove both shoes and socks even if you only have a problem with one foot. This is important as comparison of the problem foot to the good one is very helpful not to mention that your perception of a problem and ours will likely be very different. The podiatrist will ask you to expand on what you have written on your form whilst jotting down notes. At the same time they will be visually assessing the condition of your feet, looking for anything out of the ordinary and marking it on a chart.

Taking the history of any complaint is important as two problems that may look and feel the same today may well have had different causes and symptoms earlier.

Let's assume that you are attending purely for a check-up in response to reading this book or seeing the doctor. You may be surprised that the podiatrist isn't limiting their questions to your feet but is also asking about your general health and particularly any pains in your knees, hips and back. (If you've skipped to this chapter then go back and read the rest of the book to find out why there may be a link and what podiatrists can do to help).

Sensitivity tests.

Initially we will test the sensitivity to various stimuli. Don't worry: nothing will be painful. The following tests will usually be carried out:

- Monofilament.
- Neurotip.
- Tiptherm.
- Tuning fork.
- Neurothesiometer.
- Discrimination of sharp and blunt.
- Light touch.
- Proprioception.
- Reflexes.

Please note: in the Traffic Light System sensory testing is limited to the use of a monofilament to test light touch or a tuning fork to test for vibration sensation. Although giving enough helpful information for a simple screening appointment, in my view it is not comprehensive enough for most diabetics. Indeed if you are found to be at moderate or higher risk, you will be referred for more in depth tests as a matter or necessity. This is not sufficient to build up a comprehensive picture of the foot's sensory status as different nerves respond to different stimuli. For example when testing light touch there is no stimulus being applied to the nerves that sense sharp touch, temperature, or vibration. Therefore podiatrists do different tests for the different nerve types. This can be critically important as you may be able to feel the monofilament and yet unable to feel sharp sensation and so you could be at risk because you don't sense that kind damage to your skin.

Circulation tests

Assessment of your pedal arteries will determine if there are any early changes in your vascular status. There are two main arteries in the feet and as a minimum they should be palpated. This means the practitioner using their fingers to sense the pulse. By itself this is really not adequate as firstly it relies on the level of sensitivity of the practitioner's hand but also on their ability to find the pulse (almost impossible in a swollen foot).

A better assessment can be made using a Doppler of which there are various types. The most basic is one that detects the blood flow and magnifies the sound so we can hear that the blood is flowing.

Better still is a bidirectional Doppler. This is a bit smarter as it can detect which direction the blood is flowing in. Our gold standard is to use a bidirectional Doppler with the capability to print out or display a picture of what the blood is doing. We use this as it is a great way of educating our clients but is also useful for referral letters.

The bidirectional Doppler shows up if the arteries have lost their elasticity. This can be caused by smoking, age, diabetes and most commonly, high cholesterol. Unfortunately high cholesterol and diabetes often coexist and we are all getting older. Perhaps you can see now why if you are a smoker you are always being nagged by your doctor and loved ones.

Furred up arteries that have lost their elasticity can be detected fairly early on using this method and assessed for any deterioration over the years. If they have deteriorated then you can be pretty sure other arteries in the body will have done the same, such as the cardiac and brain arteries. It is for this reason that in the US health insurance companies are particularly interested in the results of feet check-ups as they can be used as a predictor of the likelihood of that person having a stroke or heart attack. (They then promptly bump up the premium!)

Capillary refill time.

If your pulses are all strong, regular and triphasic, we can confidently assume that the blood is getting into the foot. However it still needs to perfuse into the smaller capillaries. For some of us even as kids if we squeeze the colour out of our big and little toes and wait for it to come back it can take longer than the ideal three seconds. This is not an issue if our arteries are healthy but if they deteriorate it will be even harder for the blood to get its life-giving oxygen, nutrients and white blood cells to fight infection to the superficial skin.

Temperature gradient

Another useful tool is to take the skin temperature at the shin and the end of the big toe to see if there is a greater than normal gradient indicating a poor blood supply to that foot. Additionally if certain areas are hotter it may indicate infection, frictional forces against the shoe or even a Charcot joint (see Chapter 10).

Comparison of left to right is also helpful in identifying early stages of peripheral arterial disease or even partial occlusion of an artery higher up the body.

Having now established a picture of the general health of the foot it is important to check for any other issues.

Visual examination

This will look for:

- Any breaks in the skin, cuts, ulcers, etc.
- Hard skin.
- Corns.
- Verrucae.
- Fungal infection.
- Bacterial infection.
- Fissures.
- Potential skin cancer lesions.
- Bony prominences such as hammer toes or bunions.

Any of these can be unpleasant but when combined with diabetes it is even more important to keep on top of them with regular care.

Structural examination.

No foot assessment would be complete without a look into the foot structure and what further damage it may be causing both in the feet and elsewhere in the body.

The podiatrist has to predict the likelihood of what we're seeing now causing problems either elsewhere in the body or later in life. For example a foot that rolls in too much can cause the leg to twist and undue stress and wear and tear to be inflicted upon the knee. This can cause an injury at any time whilst also increasing the likelihood of more gradual problems associated with wear and tear. Later in life if your knees are damaged and worn out you will either be facing a life of inactivity due to the pain (which won't help your diabetes) or the risks of surgery to replace your knee.   ❑

The effects of Foot pronation on posture

Diagram to show how when the right foot pronates (i.e: rolls down) the whole leg will rotate inwards and the pelvis will tilt anteriorly (towards the front)
If a foot is abnormally pronating it follows that the knees and hips can be affected as well as extra strain put on the lower back

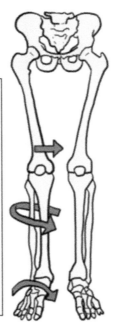
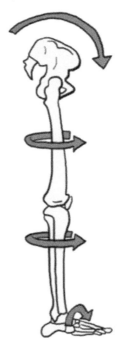

A general overview of the foot structure.

Here we are looking for prominent joints such as hammer toes, claw ❑
toes, retracted toes ,mallet toes, bunions or a plantarflexed first ray
(dropped big toe), all of which can produce areas of high pressure
and overloading.

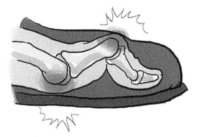

Increased angle between bones leading to:
1) Prominent areas that rub on the shoe upper.
2) An increase in pressure under the foot.

My shoes are killing me! Actually they could be!

Please turn back to Chapter 7 for illustrations of some common
deformities and the complications likely to develop because of a poor
foot structure particularly in a person with diabetes.

We also examine the gross movements such as the range of movement
at the ankle joint and particularly in the big toe joint. ❑

This can be done both while seated and also weight-bearing. If the
range of motion is diminished then the foot will not be able to
function properly and the chances are it will be compensating by ❑
moving another joint and overloading that.

Other issues may be that the deformity within a toe causes an ingrown toe
nail or even that the bone may start to grow in response to the pressure,
leading to an exostosis (the formation of new bone on the surface of a ❑
bone).

Footwear.

It is not uncommon for a person's shoes to cause problems (see
the following chapter) so your podiatrist will ask you to bring in a
selection of the shoes you wear the most and may advise a change ❑
of style or size. We are not killjoys and encourage you to wear your
special shoes occasionally so long as it is done with care. The better

you look after your feet and wear sensible shoes for your everyday life the longer you will be able to continue getting away with the ❏ ones for those special occasions. It should be stressed that ill-fitting or inappropriate shoes have contributed massively to many diabetic foot ulcers and amputations. ❏

Many people who consult me do so with issues that can be resolved quite easily for example by changing a shoe type or the way they walk with the use of an orthotic device (see following chapter) yet they choose to come ❏ back every two or three months simply because they haven't grasped what's causing the problem or because the cost puts them off.

After the initial assessment you will be advised on the most appropriate treatment plan for you. This will generally include a combination of addressing the at-risk areas and preventing further at-risk areas developing.

There is generally an overlap of aims for different treatments. For example, an orthotic insole may be made to offload an at-risk area but may also be designed to alter the foot's function and prevent further deformity and deterioration of the foot's structure. They may also be used to correct the alignment of the foot and leg thus reducing knee pain and preventing deterioration. ❏

Typically a treatment plan may include:

- Routine reduction of hard skin and management of toenails.
- Footwear advice. ❏
- Self-care advice.
- Gait analysis.
- Pressure plate or in-shoe pressure analysis.
- A biomechanical assessment.
- Accommodative or functional orthotics.
- Muscle stretching and or strengthening exercises.

Thereafter regular visits will be advised dependent on the findings. Generally, if there are no complications and a person has been advised on probable future complications, then an annual review is sufficient to reassess and note any deterioration particularly in nerve function, circulation, and foot structure.

Usually though regular visits are needed the frequency of these is determined by the scale of the problem you have and the control of your diabetes. A person may have a build-up of hard skin that requires debridement every three months while someone with a circulatory issue may require it every four weeks.

Prevention is always better than cure and in diabetic care prevention is always a top priority:

• Prevention of the deformity coming.
• Prevention of the callus forming.
• Prevention of that callus becoming extravasated.
• Prevention of that extravasation becoming a breakdown.
• Prevention of that breakdown becoming an ulcer.
• Prevention of that ulcer becoming infected.
• Prevention of that infection becoming cellulitis or bone infection.
• Prevention of that part of the foot being amputated.
• Prevention of the foot being amputated.
• Prevention of the leg being amputated.
• Prevention of the other foot and leg being amputated.
• Prevention of death.

Prevention prevention prevention! And the only way we can do that is by educating and working with you.

Sometimes the build up of hard skin becomes darker with areas of bleeding within it. This is because the pressure has built up so much that the capillaries have leaked blood into the skin. It is a warning that there is too much pressure there and is usually the precursor, if not dealt with, of an ulcer. Your podiatrist will therefore be requesting more frequent visits to prevent this deterioration which otherwise may lead to catastrophic effects. In fact **around 80% of all diabetic amputations have an ulcer as the root cause.**

If an early Charcot joint (see Chapter 10) is suspected the foot should be kept immobilised in a cast for a considerable time to maintain its shape, thus preventing new pressure points from developing which would themselves become high risk areas.

Schedule regular podiatry check-ups.

Although the majority of patients with diabetes respond well to their advice and attend regularly, some do not. Some may not have any complications yet but it is still important for them to attend their diabetic foot assessment every year. This should also be scheduled for the person who visits their podiatrist regularly for routine care as it is often hard to notice gradual changes taking place.

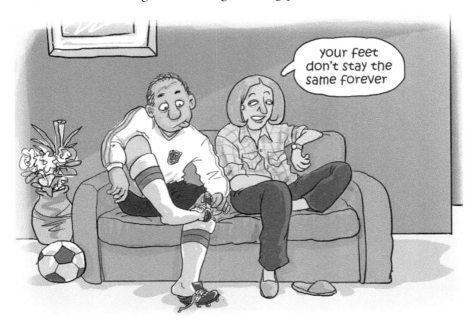

A person with diabetes would benefit from a twice yearly check; one in the summer and one in the winter. There can be weather specific conditions which need addressing in different ways.

A summer check-up may identify fungal infections which can easily deteriorate into cellulitis if they have bacterial infection superimposed on them. Clients may need to be reminded to wear sun cream to prevent a foot that has no sensation of temperature from burning or to wear supportive sandals and possibly even bespoke sandals. Then there are dry heels – they can quickly deteriorate and crack leading to potential sites of infection.

A winter check-up is more likely to look for areas of chilling where skin can die because there is no blood getting through to it. Advice can be given on how to prevent this chilling. Clients may also need to ❏ be reminded not to expose their feet to extreme temperatures. If they have temperature sensation neuropathy they shouldn't let their feet get too cold or then subsequently expose them to too much heat such as an excessively hot foot bath or hot water bottle or even by putting ❏ them too close to a fire. All these examples have led to people losing a limb because of damage to their skin and underlying tissues which then can't heal well and fall victim to infection. ❏

Staying 'Undefeeted™' should be at the forefront of your mind and I encourage you to make three solid agreements now which together ❏ should ensure you remain in the sweet spot with the least chance of ❏ developing these devastating complications of diabetes.

Make an agreement with yourself.

As a Christian I believe you are God's creation and your body is His temple. Whether you believe this or not, life is a gift and we should respect it and do our best to embrace it and live the fullest life possible. So I encourage you from this day forward to give your feet ❏ the attention they deserve.

1. Identify the risk factors and put systems in place to minimise that ❏ risk.

2. Commit to seeking help early if you notice anything unusual. ❏

3. Check regularly for any early problems with your feet – particularly if you have lost sensation – as you can't rely on feeling to tell you ❏ something is wrong.

Exercise: get into the sweet spot.

Go back through the tick boxes in this chapter and answer the questions or complete the statements below.

1. What is the most important thing that you have learned in this chapter?

....

....

....

....

2. Which main risk factor have you become aware of?

....

....

....

....

3. The one big thing I am going to start/stop doing is

....

....

....

....

If you need to break that down into several steps, please go ahead and note them below. Make sure to add the date by which you intend to achieve each of those steps.

....

....

....

....

Chapter 14:

Commit to yourself.

> *"Perchance he for whom this bell tolls may be so ill, as that he knows not it tolls for him... No man is an island, entire of itself; every man is a piece of the continent, a part of the main."*
>
> John Donne 1572-1631 Meditation Xv11.

With diabetes often it is someone else rather than yourself who becomes alarmed by changes in your foot. It is usually a professional who spots the problem (generally by chance) and often while the person with the problem has lived in blissful ignorance of it for some time. What we need is an accountability partner. This can be a loved one, spouse, child, parent or other family member.

I am aware that some of you may not have someone to fill this role and that is one good reason for joining a diabetic sweet spot group where like-minded people will be keen to help you (alternatively you could join the online group at **www.undefeeted.org/sweetspot**). With the wonders of social media and smart phones your accountability partner could be receiving photos of your feet on the other side of the world: it's not ideal but is still better than nothing.

You could use a selfie pole to take pictures of your feet if you have problems bending down. Alternatively take a photo of them in a mirror (remember you need to see the soles underneath and between the toes as well as the view you normally see of the tops of your feet). Watch the video of how to do this at **www.undefeeted.org/videos**.

Make a commitment with a team of professionals.

This agreement will differ considerably depending on the state of your feet. It may change over time if things improve or deteriorate. At a basic level it means agreeing to go for a check-up and thorough ❑ diabetic foot assessment tests every year. By the way, your team should definitely include a podiatrist!

Many of these tests can be carried out by professionals other than podiatrists such as nurses and doctors. However there's no doubt that the best level of assessment and care would be provided by a podiatrist. Our training is very thorough and many specialist issues are often overlooked by someone who hasn't done that level of training.

Your wellbeing depends on YOU.

It doesn't matter how many healthcare professionals work with you or how many loved ones keep an eye open for problems associated with your diabetes if you don't take care of yourself.

You are the person who can do most for you. If you are reading this it's either because you bought the book or someone bought it for you. Either way you are to be commended for having picked it up and got this far.

What I want more than anything is for you to put this book down and feel empowered by what you've learned. Each of you should ❑ finish the last page knowing what can go wrong with diabetic feet. ❑ More importantly, you will have gained an understanding of how at risk you are personally of future complications because of your ❑ diabetes. To get firmly and securely into the sweet spot you need to act. The chapters that follow will help you plot your course into that ❑ safe haven.

Some of you will have had recent professional assessments and have been told where you stand right now. However there is a limit to what those assessments can cover. Chapter 7 will have given you an insight into the complexity of your feet so you no longer have any excuse to see them as 'plates of meat'.

DIY care.

The Ipswich touch test, devised by Dr Gerry Rayman and his team at Ipswich hospital here in the UK (it's now been adopted by Diabetes UK and is also known as the **touch your toes test**), is a quick and simple way for you to get a warning of just how much danger you are in. It gives you an indication of how your nerves may have been affected. I'm grateful to Gerry for his explanation of how to do this test.

It should be stressed that this test is in no way meant to be a substitute for an annual foot screening appointment by a suitably trained health professional.

Touch your toes test.

- To carry it out all you need is your feet and another person to touch them.
- The other person will ask you to shut your eyes so you can't cheat and they will then touch the end of six of your toes very gently and briefly.
- Every time you feel a touch you'll tell them where you felt it.
- They should use their index finger and the touch should be as light as a feather lasting for 1-2 seconds. They should not be tempted to poke, prod, press, tap or stroke the skin.
- If you don't feel the touch on a toe, the other person should simply record that rather than pressing harder.
- Likewise, if not felt they shouldn't try again, there is no second chance.

The test should be done in the following order:

1. Right big toe.
2. Right little toe.
3. Left big toe.
4. Left little toe.
5. Right middle toe.
6. Left middle toe.

Every time the patient responds correctly put a Y on the diagram corresponding to that toe. If they did not respond put a N.

How to interpret the results

If you can feel five or six toes then your sensation is said to be normal and you should not be in any immediate danger of developing a foot problem because of a lack of sensation. You should still have your ❏ annual in-depth checks done even if you did well on this test,

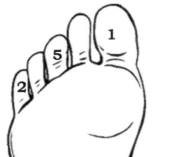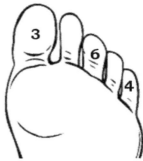

Touch your toes test - order of touching toes

If you did not feel two or more of your toes you are very likely to have reduced sensitivity and therefore may be at risk of developing a foot problem. It is then important to have a more detailed assessment by a ❏ podiatrist who will tailor your foot care plan to your needs. ❏

Get used to looking at your feet. ❏

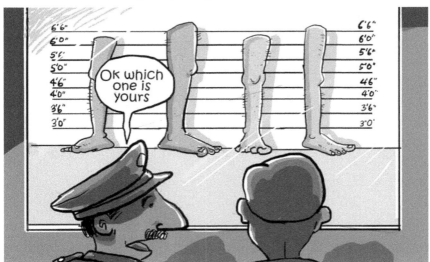

How well do you know your feet?

Get into the habit of knowing what your feet look like. The earlier complications in diabetes are noticed the better – provided that you act promptly. The earlier a problem is addressed the better the outcome is likely to be. ❏

Things you may be able to see for yourself:

- **Shoe wear (similar to tyre wear).** If it is uneven it can indicate a problem. If a shoe is too worn it can alter the way your foot ❏ functions and your gait (remember page 94).

- **Deformities** that have developed such as toes clawing, bunions or hammer toes. These and other deformities can produce bony ❏ prominences which are more likely to develop a pressure lesion.

- Check if you have **knock knees** or are bowlegged – look at ❏ yourself in a mirror.

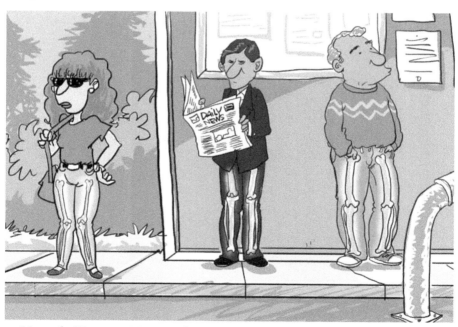

Knock Knees, Normal or Bow Legged. Which are you?

- Are your **arches too flat?** What sort of footprint is left on the ❑ bathroom floor when you step out of the bath?

Different types of foot

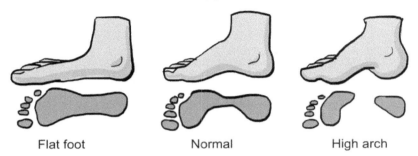

| Flat foot | Normal | High arch |

As you may be growing bored with my car analogies, another way of considering how important the feet are is to think about a building.

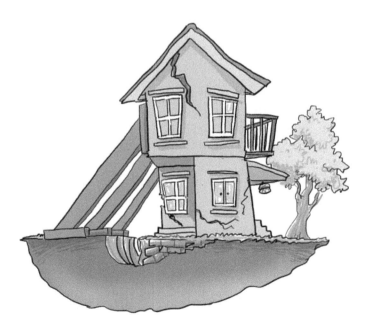

Just as poor foundations can cause a house to crack higher up, so too your feet can cause problems higher up in your body.

Insurance companies are aware that the foundations of a house are important, that's why they have a larger excess for any subsidence-related claims. They know that any signs of early subsidence should be addressed and that if it's not it is only going to get worse. A small amount of movement at foundation level can cause catastrophic effects higher up. ❏

How sure are you that your foundations, your feet, can withstand all you will expect of them over the 80 or so years you'll be standing and walking on them? In recent surveys carried out ❏
by Circle Podiatry 80% of respondents said they weren't sure. Almost the same number said they would like to find out, yet only a very small proportion acted on this.

- **How do your feet look when you are walking?** A lot of our posture and gait habits are caused by what our feet are doing because of their structure. ❏

So get a friend or partner to stand at one end of your hallway and video the way you walk with your phone. Better still do it barefoot and zoom in on the feet. Take a look, maybe your feet are collapsing inwards or pointing outwards a bit like Charlie Chaplin. You can ❏
watch some examples at **www.undefeeted.org/videos**.

- **Concentrate on your feet.** Do they ever cause any pain? ❏

Pain is supposed to be an early warning sign, not an everyday experience, yet it is not unusual for people to put up with it in their feet until it becomes unbearable. ❏

What about back, knee or hip pain? Keep a simple pain diary. You can download one from **www.undefeeted.org/resources**.

- **Do you have any inflamed areas?** These may appear red and swollen and feel hot to the touch. This may be due to infection or an inflammatory response. If you have a hot swollen painful ❏
(or painless) foot, ankle or knee get it checked out as it may be the early stages of a Charcot joint forming, which is a medical emergency that we discussed in Chapter 10.

- **Any ingrowing nails?** It's better to catch these when they're a little bit red and sore rather than waiting until they're oozing pus, 10 times more painful and are the potential cause of an amputation. ❏

- **Look out for areas of callus and corns.** They shouldn't be there and indicate too much pressure or friction. They may seem only to be a bit of a nuisance but can lead to ulcers and subsequent infection and the need for surgery or amputation. ❏

- **Watch out for dry skin.** As a person with diabetes if your skin becomes cracked, for example around the heels, it will make your foot much more susceptible to infection. ❏

- **How about infections?** ❏

  - Athletes foot is a fungal infection in the skin or nail. The earlier it's caught the better.

  - Verrucae. A verruca is a viral infection and is basically a wart on your foot. If it's on the sole of your foot (also called the plantar surface of the foot) they usually are not raised like a wart (another name for them is plantar warts). These are more of a nuisance than a danger although it is possible to get a dangerous secondary bacterial infection. Treatment usually involves killing the skin they are living on which could potentially cause a wound. Thus care should be taken and really as someone with diabetes you are best avoiding self treatments and seeing a professional. In fact most over-the-counter treatments warn ❏ that people with diabetes should not use them.

  - Bacterial problems. Any weeping area should be dealt with as a matter of urgency. If in doubt assume there is an infection and get ❏ professional help which is likely to include prophylactic antibiotics.

- Use your phone to **photograph your feet** and in a year's time compare the two photos. Are the bunions deteriorating or the toes clawing? Are the feet more swollen? Have they got dryer? Are there any new areas of hard skin or have your feet lost their hairs? ❏ Each of these changes would otherwise go unnoticed and that could mean that you miss something important. ❏

- **Get into the habit of a daily routine.** It doesn't matter which risk category you fall into, a daily routine of self-care will mean you are taking your feet and foot care seriously. Don't wait until you have ❏ developed a problem to get serious: **start today**. You can use my ❏ easy to follow five minutes a day sweet spot checklist to help you and, before you know it, it will become second nature. It is likely ❏ you will find that it is addressing some of your diabetic sweet spot targets that you have already identified earlier in the book. ❏

  I will list these in the order I work with. You can rearrange it slightly if you'd prefer. For example some people sit down to watch the 10 o'clock news every evening. It may help them to make it a part of their daily ritual to slip off their socks and slippers and spend ❏ a few moments inspecting their feet at the same time. Ladies, as masters of multi-tasking, you may be better at this than us men. People often say it's easy to attend to your feet while listening to the news just glancing up to see anything of particular interest. ❏ Please make a commitment to do the following simple checks on a daily basis.

The seven minutes a day sweet spot checklist:

- When you get home take your shoes off as soon as you get in the front door. **0 seconds (you do it anyway)**.

  Don't walk into the house with your shoes on! Not only will you ❏ bring all sorts of sources of infection from outside but also there is the possibility of treading into your home bits of grit or even glass that you have trodden on outside, only for you to tread on it later barefoot around the house (mind you, really you shouldn't be walking around the home barefoot for that very reason).

- Check the shoes' soles on the bottom and insides. **30 seconds**. Look ❏ for glass stuck in the sole and feel inside for bits of grit. If you find anything remove it there and then – don't wait until later – then if you found something, before you forget check your foot just in case the grit or glass has already caused a wound you are unaware of.

- Put on slippers or house shoes. **10 seconds**. ❏

- Later that evening shower or bathe and pay attention to your feet; ❑ wash every part of them including between the toes. **30 seconds**.

- Use a towel to dry your feet carefully. However for between the toes a safer method is to use a piece of folded up kitchen paper. ❑ It absorbs well and it will tear before your skin does (the skin between the toes can tear easily). If you have an infection on one foot and not the other (such as athletes foot) make sure to use a different piece for each foot. **30 seconds**. ❑

- If the space between your toes looks white or soggy it is because they are too moist and the air isn't getting to them. Use a cotton ❑ bud or another piece of kitchen paper with surgical spirit on it to cleanse between them. Surgical spirit will help dry the skin which will make it less susceptible to infections. Your podiatrist ❑ will advise you if you need to do this. **1 minute**.

- If your Podiatrist has okayed you to do gentle self treatments of hard skin in specific areas spend some time sanding those areas before putting cream on. Check first that your Podiatrist ❑ is ok with you doing this and has advised/shown you what to do. Generally if given the all clear you should lightly rub with medium grade sandpaper or a pumice stone.(Please note the metal cheese grater style devices, anything too course or any powered device should not be used) Remember a little often is ❑ safer than trying to remove too much at once. **2 min.**

- Apply a good specialist foot cream with a high urea content such as ❑ CCS cream or Flexitol. **2 minutes (remember not between the toes**.

- When you get out of bed in the morning put your slippers on ❑ again. **0 seconds**.

- Check inside your socks. This may seem crazy but only the other day I felt something under my big toe and on looking I found a little piece of wire had somehow got into my sock! I still don't know how that happened but I'm glad I took the time to check, I ❑ could so easily have ended up with a wound. **10 seconds**.

- Check inside your shoes again. Yes, I know you did it yesterday, but something could easily have fallen in since then, especially if you have kids or pets. I have known people to walk around all day with something in their shoe. One lady (not a diabetic) walked to the end of the garden and back in her wellies with a dead mouse in the end of the boot! **10 seconds**. ❑

Total: seven minutes per day.

Please see Chapter 14 for further advice on what you should do for yourself. This is based on your current risk category which you'll learn at your annual ❑ screening with your podiatrist (pleast see Chapters 15 and 16).

What you put your feet through.

We all like our own space and most of us would prefer not to live in a cramped house. Our feet are just the same, yet we force them to live in inappropriate houses. That's right: your choice of footwear, ❑ both shoes and hosiery (socks, tights and stockings), are what you expect your feet to live in for the best part of the day. It's a pity that many people buy them for style and fashion rather than comfort. Podiatrists will advise you to wear the most sensible shoes possible for your everyday life – then you'll probably be able to get away with those fashion shoes once in a while. ❑

As someone with diabetes it is critical that you pay attention to this advice and act accordingly. Poorly fitting footwear and unsuitable shoes contribute to the majority of foot complications in people with diabetes. You'll find a thorough list of the advice I give my diabetic ❑ clients regarding suitable footwear below.

What is the best type of shoe? ❑

It should have a strap or lace as this serves to hold the foot firmly, ensuring it doesn't slide backwards and forwards as you walk. It also ❑ gives the foot the best support. This will help prevent the foot shearing as it slides which can cause blisters and callus. The foot shearing can ❑ also cause existing callus to move as a solid mass causing trauma such as pinching and fissuring. ❑

For these reasons slip on shoes are not advisable. Slippers also provide very little support so I normally recommend house shoes also with a strap or lace. ❑

The heel height should not be more than 3 cm (1.25 inches) high. ❑

The upper should be made of a soft natural material. This serves two purposes: ❑

1. A natural material allows the foot to breathe, which is important when you consider that the average pair of feet can perspire the equivalent of half a pint of sweat every day. And infection likes a ❑ damp environment...

2. The upper should be able to stretch and adapt to fit your foot rather than being hard and unforgiving on your now delicate ❑ skin. However, I should point out that even a soft pair could easily be breaking your foot with drastic consequences. Thus the shoes may need stretching or altering to make more room for that part of the foot, particularly if it is deformed.

How to fit new shoes

1. When buying new shoes if it's possible get your foot measured. However if they say you are size 5 remember that you aren't! One shoe manufacturer's size 5 may be different to another's and different styles even from the same manufacturer will vary ❑ a bit.

2. Remember the sizing is often only referring to length so be sure to check you have enough room in the toe box both in depth and width. ❑

3. Don't forget to try both shoes on as people's feet are often different sizes and different lengths. ❑

4. Wherever possible go to the shop yourself. ❑

5. Wear the type of socks/hosiery you will wear with the new shoes. ❑

6. Your feet swell during the course of the day so, if you can, shop for shoes at the end of the day. ❑

How to get a good fit

Stand on a piece of stiff card (a cereal packet will do) with the card and your heel right up against the wall. Then either put a mark at the end of the big toes or better still get someone to draw around each foot.

If you just made a mark at the end of the big toe cut out a strip of card that long or cut out your foot's outline. You will now end up with a piece of card that is as long as your foot which you can slip into the shoe, push to the front and observe how much room is left at the back between the card and the heel counter.

Alternatively just place your shoe on top of the cut-out shape of your foot and you will probably be surprised at just what you are expecting your feet to squeeze into.

7. Try to get a pair where the footbed comes out because your podiatrist is likely to prescribe some insoles specific to your needs. ❏

8. Wear at home for a maximum of 20 minutes and check afterwards for any signs of redness or rubbing. Do this on several days, gradually increasing the time you spend wearing them. ❏

9. If you are still not sure then take the shoes along to your podiatrist. ❏

Old shoes can also cause problems:

1. If they become too worn you can end up walking unevenly and doing yourself an injury either to the foot or higher up the body. ❏

2. Too worn may well indicate the sole being too thin and thus unable to protect you from sharp objects. ❏

3. The lining may have worn and left rough edges. ❏

4. Mould growth may have occurred during storage which can lead to athletes foot. ❏

5. Your feet may no longer fit the shoes that you wore last summer. This is not just true for children, adults can be prone to swelling

and to fallen arches which will make the foot wider and elongate it. Additionally bunions and hammer toes/claw toes may have worsened over the year and so the shoe that was deep enough last year may no longer be so. ❏

Don't let that favourite pair become your downfall! If they don't fit anymore get rid of them!

Care of footwear.

1. Keep shoes clean and check inside and out for sharp objects every day. ❏

2. Change shoes daily taking out any insoles overnight so that the shoe can air. (If the insole is a prescription one don't place it on a radiator as often they are heat moulded to the shape of your foot and could distort). ❏

3. If you notice pet hairs accumulating then clean them out with the vacuum cleaner. A dog hair could get into your skin, go septic and could ultimately be the cause of an amputation – or worse. ❏

Special insoles.

There are numerous types of insoles on the market but be warned: they may not be suitable for you. Do you remember Jack from Chapter 10? The elderly gentleman who came to see me in slippers that had a tack in them? Once we had healed his wound he came back some months later with a pair of insoles that had caused a build-up of callus on his forefoot which was close to a further breakdown. He had thought he was doing something to benefit his feet, spending money on the insoles and using them. In fact he was causing a problem that could have led to an ulcer and subsequent amputation. ❏ ❏

He would have benefitted from insoles specific to his foot type and problems which I had advised him about previously. Of the many types of insoles out there I would always recommend that you seek professional advice about what is most suitable for you. ❏

That said I would like to mention two particular types which I have found helpful both for myself and for patients.

Vasyli/Armstrong.

These were designed by one of the leading orthotic producing companies after collaboration with a diabetic think tank team led by Dr David Armstrong. They can effectively address specific problem areas often experienced by the diabetic foot such as friction, pressure, and shearing forces.

"By utilising patented Glidesoft technology, this unique combination of construction and materials has been scientifically shown to reduce shear pressure in the forefoot area by 50% and dramatically reduce the onset of plantar ulcers, when compared to conventional diabetic insoles."

These insoles are made of five layers of different materials which are held together in such a way that the top surface moves with the sole of the foot thus reducing the shearing forces often found in the forefoot by up to 50%. This in turn has been shown to significantly reduce the formation of ulcers on the sole of the foot.

From the base up, the five layers are:

1. A heat mouldable EVA base that can be moulded to the shape of the person's arch.

2. A Teflon layer.

3. A shock absorbing layer.

4. A plastazote layer which self-moulds to the sole providing a soft full contact surface for the foot.

5. A constant temperature top layer which helps to prevent uneven temperature and hot spots.

These multiple properties, along with the fact that the device should be heat moulded for an optimum fit, means that they should only be fitted by an appropriate health professional such as a podiatrist.

Two other benefits of these are insulation from the plastazote layer in cold weather preventing chilling and the fact that they are quite thick which diminishes the chance of foreign bodies penetrating the shoe sole and reaching the foot.

However the multiple layers do mean they are thicker than most insoles and so appropriately deep shoes should be sourced to prevent pressure points on the tops of the feet. ❏

Liqua Care® insoles

Duncan Stang, National Co-ordinator of Diabetes in Scotland, led the research into these insoles. He said: "These insoles are particularly helpful if you have peripheral vascular disease as they are designed in such a way as to enhance the circulation within the foot allowing ❏ more oxygen to reach the tissues meaning they are less likely to break down or more likely to heal if there is already a wound present.

"They work by a viscous non-toxic liquid gel within adjoining compartments inside the insole. As the foot moves, the gel flows from one compartment to the next (and thus redistributes areas of pressure ❏ on the sole) and leads to increased small muscle activity within the feet.

"This in turn facilitates improved venous and lymphatic flow, as well as increased delivery of arterial blood to the capillary bed. Although during research the increase in oxygen in the tissues was observed as small, it is likely to be clinically significant. Moreover, the enhanced tissue oxygenation was observed after just two weeks' insole use. Given the proposed mechanism of action, it is thought that wearing the insoles for a longer period of time may be associated with an even greater improvement in tissue oxygen delivery, which will protect the ❏ foot against tissue breakdown and ulceration."

Research has also shown that Liqua Care® insoles can reduce forefoot pressure by an average of 21% as well as improving tissue oxygenation. These two effects should help prevent new and recurrent foot ❏ ulceration in people who are at risk of developing this complication of diabetes.

Two other advantages of these insoles are that they are cost-effective and not very bulky so they can often be slipped into the person's shoe without making it too tight. Care should still be taken during the wearing in process or when they are introduced to a different pair of ❏ shoes to ensure they are not causing pressure or rubbing on the upper.

One final point to note for people in the UK is that they have been proven to be so effective that they have now been included in the list of things available on prescription in this country.

Duncan Stang makes no financial gain from these insoles.

Prescription shoes.

These are made specifically for you if the foot is a shape that cannot be accommodated by a high street shoe. ❑

They cost a lot, so if you've been prescribed some you definitely need them as they aren't just given out to anyone. So make sure to wear them and don't be tempted to dabble with your old favourites or that lovely pair you saw in the shop window.

They will nearly always have moulded insoles inside which are part of ❑ the prescription and should be kept with the shoe.

Prescription orthotics

Orthotics are insole devices that address any abnormality of the foot's ❑ structure encouraging it to function in a more normal way. They should be issued only after a thorough examination of the feet and lower limbs, which allows the prescribing podiatrist to prescribe the correct devices. They are likely to differ from left to right and under ❑ no circumstances should you wear someone else's.

Broadly speaking they come in three different classes:

1. **Temporary off-the-shelf** can be adapted by the podiatrist making appropriate additions to them. ❑

2. **Semi-bespoke off-the-shelf.** These are often heat mouldable to the shape your foot (done with the foot held in a better position than its natural relaxed one) and also rely on extra pieces being ❑ stuck on.

3. **Bespoke.** These are made from a model of your foot and have the advantages of often being slimmer and a better fit to the contours ❑ of your foot. They also last considerably longer.

Orthotics have helped many people suffering from all kinds of problems such as foot, knee, hip, back, and even neck and shoulder pain. They should help prevent deformity, overloading and shearing forces, meaning that injured structures have a chance to heal whilst also preventing further damage being sustained.

Exercise: get into the sweet spot

Take a look at the tick boxes in this chapter and answer the questions or complete the statements below.

1. What is the most important thing that you have learned in this chapter?

....

....

....

....

2. Which main risk factor have you become aware of?

....

....

....

....

3. The one big thing I am going to start/stop doing is

....

....

....

....

If you need to break that down into several steps, please go ahead and note them below. Make sure to add the date by which you intend to achieve each of those steps.

....

....

....

....

Chapter 15:
Let your friends or family help.

Some people shout from the rooftops about their diabetes, cancer or other ailment while others live quietly with their condition. Who is right? It's a difficult question to answer. I feel it's down to the individual to make the choice for themselves. It does however make some sense to inform people at work or friends you dine with so they can take into account your dietary requirements. ❑

This chapter, albeit short, is important, and could make all the difference to whether a person gets into and stays safely inside the sweet spot – and indeed between having an amputation or not. Our loved ones and friends could ultimately help us make a positive impact on our life expectancy. ❑

The following verses from the Bible show the benefit of not going it alone in your walk with diabetes.

"Two are better than one,
because they have a good return for their labour:
[10] If either of them falls down,
one can help the other up.
But pity anyone who falls
and has no one to help them up.
[11] Also, if two lie down together, they will keep warm.
But how can one keep warm alone?
[12] Though one may be overpowered,
two can defend themselves.
A cord of three strands is not quickly broken.

Ecclesiastes Ch4 vs 9-12, **New International Version (NIV).**

Here King Solomon gives us God's message that two working together are better than one, a strong indication that we need others in our lives to help us and be helped by us. Have someone in your life help you defend yourself against the risks of diabetes and prevent you ❏ being overpowered by it.

The passage goes on to teach us that in fact we should include God in our relationships (a cord of three strands is not easily broken) and that if we do so we will be even stronger. It can be a powerful force for good (as can any strong friendship) especially if the last line is taken into account and we involve our creator in our lives.

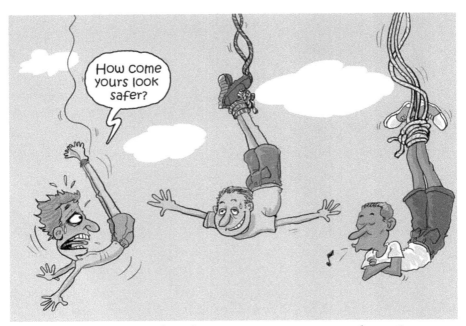

You'll be safer the more support you have!

Whilst we are on this controversial topic, I should also share my belief that as a Christian, God is able to and often does heal people and so I think it would be wrong of me not to suggest you pray for ❏ your health and for that of others and perhaps also ask others to pray for you.

Although you are the person living with the condition and are primarily responsible for your own wellbeing, friends and family should play a big part in the management of your diabetes. To that ❏ end please give some thought to who you could approach about being an accountability buddy. I detest that term and have been ❏ racking my brain for a better one. (Sweet spot sidekick maybe?) They don't have to be a family member or friend as some people feel more comfortable linking up with someone they don't know. I hope that our Undefeeted™ campaign will have small groups of people with diabetes meeting both online and on terra firma to support each ❏ other in living in the sweet spot.

Why a buddy is so important.

1. Having an accountability buddy (or trio) is a valuable asset, especially if they have diabetes as well. The two of you can really **learn from each other's experiences** and you will find when you ❏ are advising someone your own conviction will deepen.

2. **Support**. This is critical at all stages of living with diabetes if you want to remain in the sweet spot. ❏

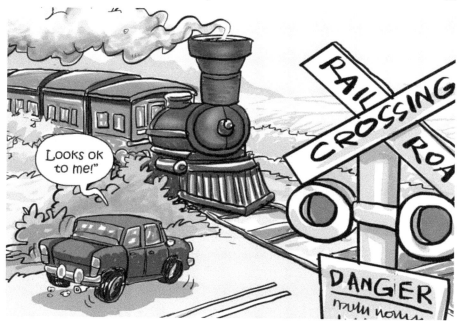

Sometimes you just don't see the danger yourself or notice the warning signs!

3. Having **a third-party view of how well you are positioned in the sweet spot**. Often we can get too comfortable and think we are okay when in fact we are in danger. ❑

4. Having a buddy who can **keep you on the straight and narrow** by: ❑

   a. Challenging you to eat better, exercise more, pay more attention to your feet, wear house shoes, put cream on etc.

   b. Encouraging you to live within the sweet spot.

   c. Praising you for doing well.

5. Your buddy can help you **be more organised**. Maybe you need help scheduling appointments for self-checks and dates to put into practice all the action points you are amassing from reading this book. ❑

6. **Practical help**:

   a. Reaching feet to care for them. ❑

   b. Cutting nails (if they've been given the okay by your podiatrist). ❑

   c. Taking shoes off. As advised earlier it's best to take them off as soon as you get through your front door. For some people this may not be practical so they run the risk of walking germs, glass or grit through the house. ❑

   d. Clearing up any broken glass or crockery. ❑

   e. Being the person's eyes. The person may well have diabetic retinopathy or just poor eyesight and can't see (or feel) what's going on with their feet. The sad truth is that the cause of a lot of the complications in a diabetic foot is also behind retinopathy and loss of sight. Not only that but in my experience when my blood sugars are high my eyesight is affected. Two years ago I took it upon myself to undertake Newcastle University's Diabetes Reversal Diet and only a short way in I became aware that my close up vision had improved to the point that I needed new glasses – yes it turned into a very ❑

expensive diet but how I enjoyed confusing the poor optician! Poor eyesight can cause a problem, for example not seeing that your spouse has moved the coffee table and splitting open your little toe. **It can mean you don't spot a problem early enough.** ❏ This is especially crucial if you have developed neuropathy. A buddy can also see if you are doing something wrong such as having your feet too close to the fire.

f. Helping with the food shopping and choosing what to eat. ❏

g. Holding you accountable to your exercise plan. ❏

h. Your friend can introduce you to **new healthy meals** and snacks. ❏

i. You can **share any targets/challenges** from your podiatrist or other health professional (or for that matter from this book) and work out an appropriate plan of action. ❏

Living with family or friends can be a bit of a double-edged sword, on the one hand it can help with your management and early detection of problems and on the other it can bring its own challenges.

Many people live alone which again comes with both advantages and disadvantages. If you are alone you know what has happened in your home (there isn't a teenage son who has broken a glass and forgotten to tell you about it). The temptation of eating pudding with the kids or those Jaffa cakes in the cupboard is removed – you shop with only yourself in mind. The family's hobbies won't pose a risk either. I enjoy ❏ working with metal to make model steam trains and am very aware that the small shards of metal that fall to the floor pose a threat to myself and my daughter.

On the other hand if you live alone you have to clear up the broken glass if you drop one, and that could be quite a dilemma if you dropped it whilst walking barefoot. ❏

If you live alone you'll have no one to check the bottom of your feet – but you can overcome this by using a mirror or taking photos. ❏

Reach out to a family member or friend who, just once a week, could visit and take a look at your feet. Ask them to hold you accountable ❏

to your wellbeing goals and advise you on what they think needs to be done.

This special person in your life will help you stay in the sweet spot. Ask them to read up on the subject and keep you up to date with the latest ideas. They can help keep you aware of just how at risk you are ❑ and finally help and hold you accountable for the actions you need to take.

If your spouse is supportive then you are at a distinct advantage as they will be sharing your habits and lifestyle with you and will know how you are behind closed doors. ❑

Set a date every year to carry out your own observations and tests: ❑

1. Comparing photos of your feet from the previous year as gradual changes in shape and structure may go unnoticed.

2. Comparing sizes, shape and colour of any moles.

3. Checking for any new areas of callus.

4. Checking for changes in skin colour or for the presence of hairs.

5. Touch the toes test. (see page 189).

6. Hot/cold test (see Chapter 13).

7. Capillary refill test (see Chapter 13).

I strongly suggest recording your results either in the **My Action Plan** section at the back of the book, or at **undefeeted.org/myactionplan** ❑ or at least in a dedicated notebook/document. Take photos in good light and from different angles. When taking photos of a mole do so ❑ with a ruler next to it to clearly show its dimensions so you can best monitor any changes year on year.

Get involved in someone else's life and don't just do it to receive. Aim to give more than you expect in return and you will usually be pleasantly surprised. Think of someone now who you can help either on by getting to know them better or, in a less involved way, by telling ❑ them about **www.undefeeted.org** or by buying them this book.

By the way don't rely on them looking it up or even starting to read the book! It is important to you now because you have just become empowered by reading a lot of helpful information. They haven't yet and are likely to be as apathetic as you were prior to learning the facts. Make a note to follow up with them by asking how they found the website or how they're getting on with the book. ❏

Exercise: get into the sweet spot.

It's that time again... Please check the tick boxes and answer the questions or complete the statements below.

1. What is the most important thing that you have learned in this chapter?

....

....

....

....

2. Which main risk factor have you become aware of?

....

....

....

....

3. The one big thing I am going to start/stop doing is

....

....

....

....

If you need to break that down into several steps, please go ahead and note them below. Make sure to add the date by which you intend to achieve each of those steps.

....

....

....

....

Chapter 16:

Commitment to a
health professional.

Making that initial commitment to yourself is vitally important. Likewise it's essential to have people in your life supporting you. Finally it's crucial to get registered for a check-up with a podiatrist who knows what they are looking for and who can detect and address any noticeable changes in between visits. They will assess and ❏ communicate your risk status.

I remember once when I parked the car with its steering on full lock and my neighbour pointed out the massive wear on the inside of the tyre. This was a real shock for me as I'd been driving on the motorway a great deal and although I'd taken the precaution of checking the tyre pressure and thought all was well, in fact there was a problem I was unaware of that could have led to a disaster. What I needed was someone to draw my attention to it and explain what it meant, what needed to be done and the consequences of not doing anything.

My mechanic friend pointed out that it was the tracking of the front wheels and that it had been going on for some time. He went on to say that it had probably had some knock-on effects elsewhere. On investigation it was clear that one of the ball joints had become excessively worn on that side. Had I been aware and dealt with the tracking earlier I would have saved a lot of money as I wouldn't have needed to replace the ball joint.

The point I want you to understand is that you may be going about your life totally oblivious to a problem within your foot and it could be a time-bomb waiting to go off .The longer you leave it the more ❏ likely it is that it will explode and the damage may well occur further up the body.

Coaches are for sports teams, not for me.

'Some people are totally uncoachable' is something I've heard a lot in the business world. They are the ones who will always have excuses and won't listen to advice. It may be that they think they know already, or that in some way the advice doesn't apply to them, or they simply feel that now isn't the time – they're too busy or too young or old or unwell. My view is that no one is uncoachable but that it may take a mindset shift for people to be willing to take on board any advice given to them. ❑

'Pride comes before a fall' is often said about arrogant people who don't listen to others – yet how often do we stop and wonder if that old saying could apply to us too? I'm afraid that most of us don't take kindly to being given instructions on how to live. Bear these words in mind when anyone (or the advice in this book) challenges your present beliefs: it may just be that you need to apply the old saying to yourself ❑ and humble yourself enough to realise you have to change your ways.

No coach knows it all though and I encourage you to get in touch with us with your questions, suggestions and tips on ways you've found to live within the sweet spot. Please feel free to bring ideas to the table either on the forum (**www.undefeeted.org/forum**), directly ❑ to myself, or to your Undefeeted™ coach if you have chosen to work with one.

Individual sporting heroes and teams have coaches to train them and keep them accountable, to make sure that they are doing what they are supposed to be doing. Business people and politicians often have ❑ influential mentors and coaches helping them set goals, keep on track and ultimately be successful in terms of business achievements and wealth creation. Most of these people have more reason to be proud and think they know it all than you and I, yet they remain open to the need for a coach and, more importantly, to what they are advising them to do.

I have a business coach to help me and in fact I have taken on a writing coach just to help get this book done. Believe me when I say that without her this book would never have been finished. In fact I thought I had nearly finished some eight months ago but she advised that I went straight back to the drawing board. She wanted me to give you a plan that would help you find your way into the sweet spot rather than the facts alone.

In fact at the moment I have four people in my life who are coaching me on how to be more successful, two of whom are concentrating on how I can give my best to you and other people with diabetes through the Undefeeted™ campaign.

Now that you've read most of the information on what can go wrong, get yourself into the zone of making a difference and make a commitment to yourself. Take excellent care of your body. Once in that zone you are one step closer to living in the sweet spot. Yes, you still have to live in the world of stress, busy lives, dodgy food and family pressures – that's why so many fail to make lasting changes.

Here at Undefeeted™ we encourage you to take your diabetes seriously and have devised three ways to intervene and help you.

1. Recorded video courses with content to help you learn how to get into and remain within the diabetic sweet spot.

2. Online and telephone coaching.

3. Bespoke one-to-one consultations and coaching tailored precisely to your needs.

The journey forwards will probably not be easy if you choose the path to success rather than the highway to Hell. But we will have podiatrists who can coach you, hold you accountable and talk you through making those life-improving and life-saving changes.

Whatever your risk it follows that controlling your diabetes, cholesterol and blood pressure, and having your feet screened every year by a suitably-trained professional, will help to reduce the risk of developing problems with your feet.

The general advice that follows, produced by the Scottish Diabetes Foot Action Group (SDFAG), is dependent on how at risk you are based on the Traffic Light System outlined back in Chapter 13.

(The leaflets produced by SDFAG can be downloaded at **http://www.diabetesinscotland.org.uk/Publications.aspx?catId=2**).

First of all though **a word about smoking**. If you smoke you are strongly advised to stop. Smoking affects your circulation and heightens your risk in any of the following categories. It can be the ❏ difference between needing an amputation and having to be pushed around the park in a wheelchair or being able to stay on your feet doing the things you enjoy with those you love. ❏

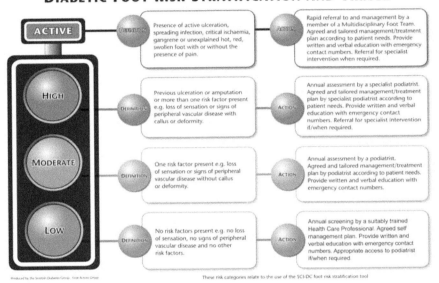

DIABETIC FOOT RISK STRATIFICATION AND TRIAGE

Low risk.

You have been screened and informed you are at low risk. If you follow the simple advice below you should be able to carry out your own foot care unless you develop a specific problem. As your feet are ❏ in good condition, you may not need regular podiatry treatment.

* You should check your feet every day for any blisters, breaks in the skin, pain, or any signs of infection such as swelling, heat or redness. ❏
* You should wash your feet every day in warm water and with a mild soap. Rinse them thoroughly and dry them carefully,

especially between the toes. Do not soak your feet as this can damage your skin. ❏

- Moisturise your feet every day if your skin is dry, avoiding the areas between your toes. ❏

- Cut or file your toenails regularly, following the curve of the end of your toe. Use a nail file to make sure that there are no sharp edges which could press into the next toe. Do not cut down the ❏ sides of your nails as you may create a 'spike' of nail which could result in an ingrown toenail.

- You should change your socks, stockings or tights every day. ❏ They should not have bulky seams and the tops should not be elasticated.

- Avoid walking barefoot. If you walk barefoot you risk injuring your feet by stubbing your toes and standing on sharp objects which can damage the skin. ❏

- Check the bottom of your shoes before putting them on to make sure that nothing sharp, such as a pin, nail or glass, has pierced the outer sole. Also, run your hand inside each shoe to check that ❏ no small objects such as small stones have fallen in.

- Ill-fitting shoes are a common cause of irritation or damage to feet. The professional who screened your feet may give you advice ❏ about the shoes you are wearing and about buying new shoes.

- If you check your feet and discover any breaks in the skin, minor cuts or blisters, you should cover them with a sterile dressing ❏ and check them every day. Do not burst blisters. If the problems do not heal within a few days, or if you notice any signs of infection (swelling, heat, redness or pain), contact your podiatry department or doctor.

- Do not use over-the-counter corn remedies. They are not ❏ recommended for anyone with diabetes as they can cause damage to the skin that could create problems. If you discover any problems with your feet, contact your local podiatry department or doctor for advice.

- Have your local podiatry department or doctor's phone number saved on your phone so you can easily and quickly access them if needed. ❏

Moderate/Increased risk.

Your screening and assessment have shown that there is an increased risk that you will develop foot ulcers. Your podiatrist will inform you which of the following risk factors you have: you have lost some feeling in your feet; the circulation in your feet is reduced; you have hard skin on your feet; the shape of your foot has changed; your ❑ vision is impaired; or you cannot look after your feet yourself.

As your feet are at an increased risk of developing ulcers, you will need to take extra care of them. You may need treatment by a podiatrist or podiatry technician. ❑

If you follow the advice and information below, it will help you to take care of your feet between visits to your podiatrist. Hopefully it will help to reduce problems in the future. ❑

- You should check your feet every day for any blisters, breaks in the skin, pain or any signs of infection such as swelling, heat or redness. ❑ If you cannot do this yourself, ask your partner or carer to help you. If you find any of these, you should contact your podiatry department or doctor immediately. If you discover any breaks in the skin, minor cuts or blisters, cover them with a sterile dressing. Do not burst blisters, hard skin or corns. Do not attempt to remove ❑ hard skin or corns yourself. Your podiatrist will provide treatment and advice where necessary.
- Have your local podiatry department or doctor's phone number saved on your phone so you can easily and quickly access it if needed. ❑
- You should wash your feet every day in warm water and with a mild soap. Rinse them thoroughly and dry them carefully, especially between the toes. Do not soak your feet as this can ❑ damage your skin. Because of your diabetes, you may not be able to feel hot and cold very well. You should test the temperature of the water with your elbow, or ask someone else to test the temperature for you. ❑
- If your skin is dry, apply a moisturising cream every day avoiding the areas between your toes. ❑

- Cut or file your toenails regularly, following the curve of the end of your toe. Use a nail file to make sure there are no sharp edges, which could press into the next toe. Do not cut down the sides ❑ of your nails as you may create a 'spike' of nail which could result in an ingrown toenail.

- You should change your socks, stockings or tights every day. ❑ They should not have bulky seams and the tops should not be elasticated.

- Avoid walking barefoot because you risk injuring your feet by stubbing your toes and standing on sharp objects which can damage the skin. ❑

- Check the bottom of your shoes before putting them on to make sure that nothing sharp, such as a pin, nail or glass, has pierced the outer sole. Also, run your hand inside each shoe to check that ❑ no small objects such as small stones have fallen inside.

- Ill-fitting shoes are a common cause of irritation or damage to feet. The podiatrist who assessed your feet may give you advice ❑ about the shoes you are wearing and advise you on buying new shoes. They may suggest that you are measured for special shoes you can get on prescription.

- Never use over-the-counter corn remedies. They are not recommended for anyone with diabetes as they can damage the skin and create ulcers. ❑

- Avoid high or low temperatures. If your feet are cold, wear socks. Never sit with your feet in front of the fire to warm them up. Always remove hot water bottles or heating pads from your bed ❑ before getting into it.

- If you discover any problems with your feet, immediately contact your local podiatry department or doctor for advice. ❑

High risk.

Your screening and assessment have shown that there is a high risk that you will develop foot ulcers. Your podiatrist will inform you which of the following risk factors you have: you have lost some feeling in your feet; the circulation in your feet is reduced; you have hard skin on your feet; the shape of your feet has changed; your vision is impaired; ❑ you cannot look after your feet yourself; you have had ulcers before; or you have had an amputation.

As your feet are at high risk, you will need to take extra care of them. You will need regular treatment by a podiatrist. ❑

If you follow the advice and information below it will help you to take care of your feet between visits to your podiatrist. Hopefully this will reduce any problems in the future.

- You should check your feet every day for any blisters, breaks in the skin, pain or any signs of infection such as swelling, heat or ❑ redness. If you cannot do this yourself, ask your partner or carer to help you. If you find any of these you should immediately contact your podiatry department or doctor. If you check your feet and discover any breaks in the skin, minor cuts or blisters; ❑ cover them with a sterile dressing. Do not burst blisters. Do not attempt to remove hard skin or corns yourself. Your podiatrist ❑ will provide treatment and advice where necessary.
- If these people are not available and there is no sign of healing after ❑ one day, go to your local accident and emergency department.
- Have your local podiatry department or doctor's phone number saved on your phone so you can easily and quickly access them ❑ if needed.
- You should wash your feet every day in warm water and with a mild soap. Rinse them thoroughly and dry them carefully, especially between the toes. Do not soak your feet as this can ❑ damage your skin. Because of your diabetes, you may not be able to feel hot and cold very well. You should test the temperature of the water with your elbow, or ask someone else to test the ❑ temperature for you.

- If your skin is dry, apply a moisturising cream every day avoiding the areas between your toes. ❑

- Do not cut your toenails unless your podiatrist advises you to. If they do then cut or file them regularly, following the curve of the end of your toe. Use a nail file to make sure that there are ❑ no sharp edges, which could press into the next toe. Do not cut down the sides of your nails as you may create a 'spike' of nail which could result in an ingrown toenail. ❑

- You should change your socks, stockings or tights every day. They should not have bulky seams and the tops should not be elasticated. ❑

- Avoid walking barefoot because you risk injuring your feet by stubbing your toes and standing on sharp objects which can damage the skin.

- Check the bottom of your shoes before putting them on to make sure that nothing sharp, such as a pin, nail or glass, has pierced ❑ the outer sole. Also, run your hand inside each shoe to check that no objects, such as small stones, have fallen in.

- Ill-fitting shoes are a common cause of irritation or damage to feet. The podiatrist who assessed your feet may give you advice about the shoes you are wearing and advise you on buying new ❑ shoes. They may suggest that you are measured for special shoes you can get on prescription.

- Never use over-the-counter corn remedies. They are not recommended for anyone with diabetes as they can damage the skin and create ulcers. ❑

- Avoid high or low temperatures. If your feet are cold, wear socks. Never sit with your feet in front of the fire to warm them up. Always remove hot water bottles or heating pads from your bed before getting into it. ❑

- If you discover any problems with your feet, immediately contact your local podiatry department or doctor for advice.

- If you have been supplied with shoes, they will have been made to ❑ a prescription. You should follow the instructions your podiatrist or orthotist (the person who made the shoes). These should be the only shoes you wear. Shoes will normally be prescribed with insoles. These are an important part of your shoes and you should only remove them if your orthotist or podiatrist advises you to. Whoever provided your shoes will carry out all repairs or alterations to make sure that they match your prescription.

- Do not attempt to remove hard skin or corns yourself. Your podiatrist will provide treatment and advice where necessary. ❑

- If you have had an ulcer before, or an amputation, you are at high risk of developing more ulcers. If you look after your feet carefully, with the help of a podiatrist, you will reduce the risk of more problems. ❑

Active foot disease.

You have a diabetic foot ulcer. This means an area of skin has broken down and the tissue under it is now exposed. ❑

A foot ulcer can become infected and the infection may become severe. It is important that you look after your foot ulcer to prevent ❑ infection occurring.

As you have a diabetic foot ulcer, you will need regular podiatry treatment. Your podiatrist will draw up a treatment plan for you to meet your needs. ❑

Diabetic foot ulcers are sometimes hidden beneath hard skin and can gather dead tissue around them. The podiatrist will need to remove this to help your ulcer heal. This can cause the ulcer to bleed a little and ❑ often it looks larger and worse than it was before so please remember the dead tissue had to be removed. This is completely normal. **Do not try to treat the ulcer yourself.** ❑

1. Do not touch the dressing unless you have been trained how to remove and replace it and you have suitable dressings to replace ❑ the one you are changing.

2. Do not get the dressing wet as it may prevent healing or allow bacteria to enter the ulcer. This will cause more problems. Your podiatrist may be able to supply you with a dressing protector to keep the ❑ dressing dry, or they may give you a form to take to your doctor to get a dressing protector on prescription. The dressing protector will

allow you to bathe or shower safely while keeping your dressing dry. ❑
For more information on this topic visit **www.undefeeted.org**.

3. Continue to check your feet every day for any other problem areas
or danger signs. Don't just look after the bad one – check the good
one too. ❑

4. **You should pay close attention to any of the following danger
signs when checking your feet:** ❑

   a. Is there any new pain or throbbing? ❑

   b. Does your foot feel hotter than usual? ❑

   c. Are there any new areas of redness, inflammation or swelling? ❑

   d. Is there any discharge? ❑

   e. Does your foot smell different? ❑

   f. Do you have any flu-like symptoms? ❑

5. If your skin is dry moisturise the area surrounding the wound
every day, avoiding areas of broken skin and between your toes. ❑

6. Avoid any unnecessary standing or walking. A wound cannot heal
if it is constantly under pressure. Rest as much as possible and
keep your foot up to help it heal. Use anything your podiatrist ❑
recommends or gives you to relieve pressure on your foot.

7. You may be asked to wear a cast (a device to relieve pressure) or a
special shoe until your ulcer has healed. You should not wear any
other footwear until your podiatrist tells you that you can wear ❑
your own shoes again.

8. Always attend your appointments to have your ulcer treated. You
may need regular appointments until the wound has healed. Your
appointment may be with a district nurse, a treatment room nurse ❑
or your podiatrist.

9. You will be given antibiotics if there are signs of infection in the wound or ❑
in the nearby tissue. Report any problems you have with the antibiotics,
such as rashes, nausea or diarrhoea, to the person who prescribed them ❑

for you. If this person is not available contact your doctor immediately. Do not stop taking your antibiotics unless the person treating you or your doctor tells you to do so. Make sure you have enough antibiotics to finish the course so your treatment isn't interrupted. ❏

10. Sometimes, if the infection is spreading, you may need to go to hospital. Here you would have antibiotics put straight into your bloodstream to treat the infection quickly. On admittance ❏ to hospital you and your wound will be assessed so that you have the most appropriate treatment plan in place. You may need a small operation to clean out the wound.

11. If an infection is very severe, an amputation may be needed to save the healthy parts of the foot. ❏

12. If your circulation is reduced, you may need a small operation to increase blood supply to the ulcerated area.
❏

13. If you discover any more problems, or if you are concerned about the treatment of your foot ulcer, immediately contact your local podiatry department or doctor for advice.

If you are in the active foot disease category then the multidisciplinary foot protection team will need to classify your wound. There are many different classification systems for diabetic wounds worldwide. One I have looked into recently I believe is the most appropriate and will probably be adopted in many more countries than its place of origin, ❏ the USA. I'll describe it briefly not because it's being used everywhere but to give you an idea of the sorts of things that your diabetic team have to take into consideration in the event of you having a foot attack/ulcer/wound that threatens your lower limb with amputation.

The WIFI system.

The WIFI (Wound, ischemia, foot infection) system was devised by Joseph Mills and David Armstrong of SALSA (Southern Arizona Limb Salvage Alliance).

If you present with a lower limb with a wound and/or poor circulation and/or infection then your limb is said to be threatened ❏ or at heightened risk of amputation.

It is important for the diabetic foot protection team to be able to classify your wound properly for the following reasons.

1. So that each member of the team understands what the others are saying (because the whole team needs to sing from the same song sheet). For example a diabetes consultant will be able to ❏ communicate the level of risk to a vascular surgeon or podiatrist.

2. Having a good classification allows the team to plan and implement an appropriate treatment plan based on facts. ❏

3. It gives the team an idea of the most likely prognosis or outcome so you too can be informed of what may need to happen. ❏

The WIFI system gives your limb a score based on:

-   Wound appearance.
-   Level of ischemia.
-   Presence/extent of infection.

A WIFI score is given for each of these categories in the following way: 0=none; 1= mild; 2=moderate; 3=severe.

Let's take a look at how a wound could score:

Wound appearance. Diabetic wounds can very quickly become deep with lots of dead tissue so that on the surface it looks small but below can be very extensive. Wounds are scored as follows:

0 = No ulcer and no gangrene.

1 = Shallow ulcer on leg or foot or deeper ulcer exposing bone on one or two toes and no gangrene.

2 = Deeper ulcer with exposed bone, joints or tendons or shallow heel ulcer not reaching bone. Gangrene limited to toes.

3 = Extensive deep ulcer to bone in forefoot and/or mid foot and/or heel and extensive gangrene to forefoot and/or mid foot and/or deep necrosis of heel including bone.

Ischemia.

The chances of a wound healing are directly linked to the blood supply as healing requires nutrients and oxygen – the body's healing process relies on a healthy blood supply. So the second score relates to your circulatory status or level of ischemia.

The ABI test.

The grade for ischemia is determined by either an ankle brachial index (ABI) reading as described in Chapter10 or the toes' blood pressure (tp).

An ABI is the difference between the blood pressure at the ankle and at the arm. The readings are taken with the person lying relaxed on a couch having rested for a while. The ABI is then calculated by dividing the highest of the blood pressures at your ankles by the higher of the two blood pressures at your arms. The resultant number is your ABI and can indicate how bad your peripheral arterial disease (PAD) is.

The readings are broken down and interpreted as follows:

1. **A reading of between 1.0 -1.4** means you probably don't have any PAD.

2. **A reading of between 0.9-0.99** suggests you may have some early narrowing of the arteries in your legs which should be monitored.

3. **A reading of between0.8-0.89** indicates that you are in the early stages of developing PAD which may need some lifestyle changes and/or medication.

4. **A reading of between 0.5-0.79** is indicative of more serious PAD. By this stage you are probably beginning to notice symptoms such as pains in your legs or buttocks when you have walked for a certain distance.

5. **A reading of below 0.5** is found if there is serious PAD and you are likely to be in pain even when resting. This is called rest pain.

6. You may be thinking that **a reading of 1.4** would be good. However if above 1.4, it is a sign that the arteries are already hardened and not able to be compressed. This is particularly relevant in a person with diabetes.

The toe pressure is carried out in the same way but as the name suggests instead of the arm and the ankle it is the arm and the big toe that are compared.

If the arteries are calcified then transcutaneous oxygen levels are used (Tcpo2). Again the grades are from 0 to 3 with 0 being no ischemia and 3 being severe ischemia.

Foot infection.

Last but definitely not least, infection is the big game changer which, when present, can cause speedy and extreme devastation. It is graded as follows:

0 = No infection present.

1 = Mild Infection present as defined by at least two of the following: local swelling; redness around the wound (between 0.5 cm-2 cm); local tenderness or pain; local warmth; thick pus discharge. The infection should only involve skin and subcutaneous tissue, nothing deeper and with no systemic signs.

2 = Moderate infection present as described above but with redness spreading further than 2 cm around the wound and involving deeper structures such as bone, tendon, abscess, joints or fascia. There should be no systemic signs of infection.

3 = Severe infection present with signs as above but also with indications of systemic inflammatory response syndrome i.e. at least two of the following present:

- Temperature more than 38 or less than 36 degrees Celsius.

- Heart rate more than 90 beats per minute.

- Respiratory rate more than 20 breaths per minute.

- White blood cell count of more than 12,000 or less than 4000.

If this book hasn't motivated you to get into the sweet spot then I hope that reading about the devastation that can so easily become a reality will scare you into ensuring you do your very best to look after yourself. ❏

Hospitalisation.

Problems like those described above require hospitalisation. In this case the focus will be on the foot, but often if a person goes into hospital for other problems the feet can be overlooked. In fact it is not unheard of for someone to be admitted because of their fever and the foot not to be looked at even though a wound there is the source of the problem.

Additionally there may be separate issues on the feet that need addressing and indeed the period in hospital itself can cause major problems due to pressure sores developing.   ❑

These problems, and research done by Dr Gerry Rayman, have led to Duncan Stang and his team developing a simple three-step programme which is being used to safeguard in-patients against foot problems either worsening or even being caused whilst in hospital.   ❑

This three-step assessment has been dubbed as CPR for diabetic feet.

CPR for feet.

C stands for Check: ❑

- Is there an ulcer or gangrene present?

- Is there neuropathy present?

- Is action required?

P stands for Protect feet if at risk due to: ❑

- Neuropathy.

- Previous ulceration or amputation.

- Bed bound or fragile skin.

R stands for Refer: ❑

- Refer all patients to the diabetic foot team or podiatry if they have an ulcer, gangrene or other major concern.

The beauty of this simple test is that it can be done very quickly and it has been shown to prevent problems and bring the average stay in hospital for people with diabetes down by an average of nine days, but that depends on whether the Protect and Refer aspects take place and happen at the right time. CPR should be carried out on initial ❏ admission and thereafter at regular intervals.

Protection of the feet may include putting a cradle over the foot of the bed to relieve pressure from the bedclothes. It should include a pressure relieving device for the heels for anyone who is bed bound because the heels are particularly prone to bed pressure sores and subsequent ulceration and infection, which can lead to amputation. ❏

My view is that this simple yet cutting edge advice will save many unnecessary wounds and amputations. I believe it should also be introduced as a weekly check for people with diabetes who live in residential or nursing homes and indeed if bed- or chair-bound at home. ❏

A final word for carers.

It is the responsibility of carers, nurses and loved ones to know the risks and signs and become the person's eyes carrying out frequent visual checks, insisting on and providing appropriate protection and timely correct referral which together can literally save the life of the ❏ person with diabetes you love or care for.

If you have just stumbled across this page or indeed have a carer looking after you then please encourage them to read this book so they get the knowledge they need to help you remain in the diabetic ❏ sweet spot even when it may be beyond your ability to do it for yourself.

Exercise: get into the sweet spot.

Go back through the tick boxes in this chapter and answer the questions or complete the statements below.

1. What is the most important thing that you have learned in this chapter?

....

....

....

2. Which main risk factor have you become aware of?

....

....

....

3. The one big thing I am going to start/stop doing is

....

....

....

If you need to break that down into several steps, please go ahead and note them below. Make sure to add the date by which you intend to achieve each of those steps.

....

....

....

Well done! You have almost reached the end of the book. I hope you've worked through each of the exercises... If not, there's no time like the present to begin. If you have completed all of the exercises, read on for further advice on how you can reach and remain within the diabetic sweet spot.

Chapter 17:
Your Personal Action Plan.

So you've made it all the way through the book. Give yourself a pat on the back for keeping going but realise that this is only the beginning of the rest of your life. I've tried to make it as simple as I can for you to live safely in the sweet spot but it's down to you now. How serious are you about keeping going over the long term? Take a look at the list you made in Chapter 4 and see which attitudes are most likely to derail you – forewarned is forearmed.

> *"At the beginning of any task, more than anything else, your attitude will affect its successful outcome."*
>
> Jeffrey Gitomer.

Whatever your age and whether you're type 1 or 2, understand that for you to be able to accomplish what you want to achieve with your feet (remember the dreams on your timeline in Chapter 4?) you need to address all the things you ticked throughout the book. That way you will understand all your new learnings, you will be in a better position to take on board the risk YOU are at, and of course you will know what actions to take.

Today you stand at a junction and you have two roads in front of you: the highway to unhealthiness (because discipline is such hard work...) or the Longevity Lane (which is harder, more challenging and often a lonelier route).

My biggest fear, based on my own knowledge of living with diabetes and experiences with individual clients, is that the enthusiasm you have now will diminish once you get back to your busy life. And the next time your feet give you a wake-up call it's likely to be a complication that could easily lead to amputation of your foot or leg.

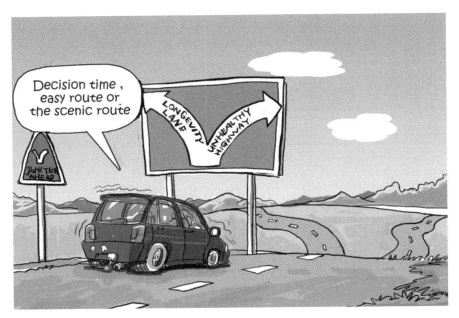

Choose wisely the directions you take in life!

Your task may at first seem daunting but if you follow the Undefeeted™ plan of tackling one action (plus the knowledge and risk associated with it) per chapter per month, then in six months you will be embedded in the sweet spot with newly formed habits replacing all those bad ones you had before.

Put this book down with the attitude that you are going to work through all the things you've learned and incorporate them into your life. Then you will have the best chance of a successful outcome.

You will have learned a lot just by reading but only a small amount will have sunk in and only a fraction is likely to be incorporated into your daily life.

What I want you to do now is plan your successful outcome by making a commitment to address one of the actions from each chapter every month over the next six months. There's no point emulating the hare and doing too much too quickly, losing interest or burning out. With that approach, you'll be lucky to cross the finish line at all and the chances are you'll be limping rather than running if you do manage to get there.

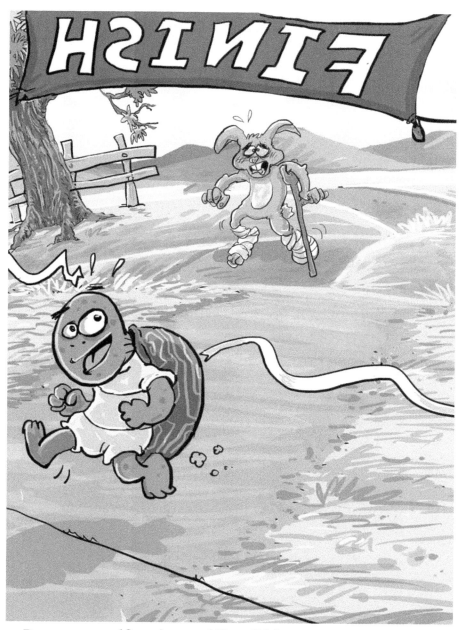

Pace yourself and your life will be turtaly awesome!

Big sweets first.

Imagine for a minute that two children are given a jar each. They are told they can have any sweets that fit in their jar. They are each allowed seven big sweets and as many smaller ones as they can fit in. The first child grabs as many small sweets as possible before realising that four of the big ones won't fit in. He has to miss out on some of his favourite sweets.

The other child also likes the big ones best and decides to put those in first and pack the small sweets around the big ones. When they count them later the jar with the seven big sweets also contains the most little ones. I learned this principle from my business coach some years ago and it is so true. At the end of a coaching session I'd have a list of all the things that needed doing and would invariably tackle one of the smaller and easier ones first, maybe leaving a harder, more time-consuming and important job until later – with the result that the latter often wouldn't get done at all.

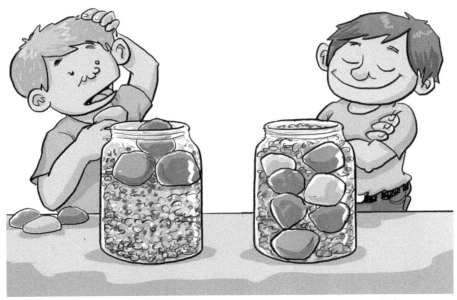

Know your 'BIG sweets' and get them sorted first.

So do the big ones first and then get on with the small ones. That way you are better placed to get more done. Also the most important ones get done first just as the second child in our example prioritised the seven big sweets before tipping in the little ones.

I would like you to apply this big sweet theory to your sweet spot exercises. Please go back through the book right now. You should have ticks on each page pertaining to things you felt you needed to learn, take on board or act upon. Hopefully you will have prioritised them in the sweet spot exercise at the end of that chapter. Some of those may have been obvious and easy to implement and you may have already addressed them satisfactorily. However I suspect you are probably still left with a potentially intimidating to-do list (or not-to-do list).

If you haven't done the exercises yet, go back and do them now. If you have been doing the exercises, I hope you've chosen to focus on the 'big sweets' (i.e. the most important/most daunting aspects). Do this for each chapter and then – either in a notebook or online at **www.undefeeted. org/myactionplan** – list all the number ones. There are also pages at the end of this chapter to help you with this. These are the target changes you are going to make over the next two to six months. It is said that it takes 66 days to create good habits[4] so spend that time ensuring you build positive new habits while ditching the bad ones.

The online resources are the ideal way to manage your own plan as they send you reminders to help keep you on track and there are a host of other useful tools for you to experiment with too.

By the end of the first month you will be well on the way to making that new action into a habit and should feel ready to move on to the next learning and associated action point. Keep going, and in six months time, you could be in the sweet spot and in a much safer position regarding not only your feet but also your eyes, kidneys and cardiovascular risk.

---

[4] Phillippa Lally, a health psychology researcher at University College London, said in her report 'How are habits formed: modelling habit formation in the real world' that 66 days is an average. It can take anywhere from 18 to 254 days for people to form a new habit. It depends on the person, their behaviour and their circumstances. The article was published in the European Journal of Social Psychology in October 2010.

I'm going to make a wild guess that some of you may have got to this point without writing anything on the previous pages. Please go back, reread and prioritise your learnings and needs so that going forward you will get the maximum value from this book.

Next steps into the sweet spot.

Once you have identified what you need to change please do the following:

1. Choose and approach an accountability buddy (or maybe two – one at home and one at work).

2. Find and contact a local sweet spot group or join the Undefeated™ online forum (**www.undefeeted.org/forum**).

3. Set reminders on your phone for each of the next six months (or list them in your diary) to ensure you know when you're due to start that month's new group of actions.

4. Alternatively you can tell us at Undefeeted™ when you are starting month one and we will send you a reminder at the end of each month (**www.undefeeted.org/remindme**).

5. Consider joining the live online class/teleseminar at **www.undefeeted. org/letsgetonline**.

6. Think about appointing an online mentor/coach to help you maximise the effectiveness of your commitment to getting into the sweet spot. Go to **www.undefeeted.org/coaching** for more information.

7. Consider working in clinic on a one-to-one basis with one of Undefeeted™'s preferred practitioners for a treatment plan tailored precisely to you (**www.undefeeted.org/coaching**).

At the end of this chapter you'll find three pages for each of the next six months. Today just fill out the first month. You will see several questions and a space to write your answers based on the sweet spot exercises you did at the end of each chapter.

At the end of the month revisit the chapter's tick boxes and choose the actions for month two (still sticking with the 'big sweets first' principle).

Give yourself prompts until the new habits become second nature, such as a Post-It note near your shoes reminding you to check them. Use whatever works best for you to remind you of the various things you are introducing or trying to quit in your life.

Please for your own sake take the right action for you. If at any point you need help then please get in touch with us. We'd also love to hear any stories you may have about your journey with diabetes as it may just be that your experience could help someone else overcome a problem or even avoid something as serious as an amputation.

I hope you've enjoyed becoming enlightened about just how amazing your feet are and have learned a ton of things about how to stay on a strong footing. I wish you the best of success on the rest of your life's journey: let's stay Undefeeted™ together.

Month 1.

Chapter 2: Are your feet killing you?

Knowledge: ....

Risk factor: ....

Action: ....

Chapter 3: Knowledge is power.

Knowledge: ....

Risk factor: ....

Action: ....

Chapter 4: Change your mindset, change your life.

Knowledge: ....

Risk factor: ....

Action: ....

Chapter 5: Time for action.

Knowledge: ....

Risk factor: ....

Action: ....

Chapter 6: Why your foot is a fortress.

Knowledge: ....

Risk factor: ....

Action: ....

Chapter 7: Foot structure and deformity.

Knowledge: ....

Risk factor: ....

Action: ....

Chapter 8: Healing rate.

Knowledge: ....

Risk factor: ....

Action: ....

Chapter 9: Circulation.

Knowledge: ....

Risk factor: ....

Action: ....

Chapter 10: Neuropathy – how is your dashboard?

Knowledge: ....

Risk factor: ....

Action: ....

Chapter 11: Infection.

Knowledge: ....

Risk factor: ....

Action: ....

Chapter 12: Be on guard.

Knowledge: ....

Risk factor: ....

Action: ....

Introduction to Part Three: Know where you stand.

Knowledge: ....

Risk factor: ....

Action: ....

Chapter 13: The foot MOT.

Knowledge: ....

Risk factor: ....

Action: ....

Chapter 14: Commit to yourself.

Knowledge: ....

Risk factor: ....

Action: ....

Chapter 15: Let your friends or family help.

Knowledge: ....

Risk factor: ....

Action: ....

Chapter 16: Commitment to a health professional.

Knowledge: ....

Risk factor: ....

Action: ....

Month 2.

Chapter 2: Are your feet killing you?

Knowledge: ....

Risk factor: ....

Action: ....

Chapter 3: Knowledge is power.

Knowledge: ....

Risk factor: ....

Action: ....

Chapter 4: Change your mindset, change your life.

Knowledge: ....

Risk factor: ....

Action: ....

Chapter 5: Time for action.

Knowledge: ....

Risk factor: ....

Action: ....

Chapter 6: Why your foot is a fortress.

Knowledge: ....

Risk factor: ....

Action: ....

Chapter 7: Foot structure and deformity.

Knowledge: ....

Risk factor: ....

Action: ....

Chapter 8: Healing rate.

Knowledge: ....

Risk factor: ....

Action: ....

Chapter 9: Circulation.

Knowledge: ....

Risk factor: ....

Action: ....

Chapter 10: Neuropathy – how is your dashboard?

Knowledge: ....

Risk factor: ....

Action: ....

Chapter 11: Infection.

Knowledge: ....

Risk factor: ....

Action: ....

Chapter 12: Be on guard.

Knowledge: ....

Risk factor: ....

Action: ....

Introduction to Part Three: Know where you stand.

Knowledge: ....

Risk factor: ....

Action: ....

Chapter 13: The foot MOT.

Knowledge: ....

Risk factor: ....

Action: ....

Chapter 14: Commit to yourself.

Knowledge: ....

Risk factor: ....

Action: ....

Chapter 15: Let your friends or family help.

Knowledge: ....

Risk factor: ....

Action: ....

Chapter 16: Commitment to a health professional.

Knowledge: ....

Risk factor: ....

Action: ....

Month 3.

Chapter 2: Are your feet killing you?

Knowledge: ....

Risk factor: ....

Action: ....

Chapter 3: Knowledge is power.

Knowledge: ....

Risk factor: ....

Action: ....

Chapter 4: Change your mindset, change your life.

Knowledge: ....

Risk factor: ....

Action: ....

Chapter 5: Time for action.

Knowledge: ....

Risk factor: ....

Action: ....

Chapter 6: Why your foot is a fortress.

Knowledge: ....

Risk factor: ....

Action: ....

Chapter 7: Foot structure and deformity.

Knowledge: ....

Risk factor: ....

Action: ....

Chapter 8: Healing rate.

Knowledge: ....

Risk factor: ....

Action: ....

Chapter 9: Circulation.

Knowledge: ....

Risk factor: ....

Action: ....

Chapter 10: Neuropathy – how is your dashboard?

Knowledge: ....

Risk factor: ....

Action: ....

Chapter 11: Infection.

Knowledge: ....

Risk factor: ....

Action: ....

Chapter 12: Be on guard.

Knowledge: ....

Risk factor: ....

Action: ....

Introduction to Part Three: Know where you stand.

Knowledge: ....

Risk factor: ....

Action: ....

Chapter 13: The foot MOT.

Knowledge: ....

Risk factor: ....

Action: ....

Chapter 14: Commit to yourself.

Knowledge: ....

Risk factor: ....

Action: ....

Chapter 15: Let your friends or family help.

Knowledge: ....

Risk factor: ....

Action: ....

Chapter 16: Commitment to a health professional.

Knowledge: ....

Risk factor: ....

Action: ....

Month 4.

Chapter 2: Are your feet killing you?

Knowledge: ....

Risk factor: ....

Action: ....

Chapter 3: Knowledge is power.

Knowledge: ....

Risk factor: ....

Action: ....

Chapter 4: Change your mindset, change your life.

Knowledge: ....

Risk factor: ....

Action: ....

Chapter 5: Time for action.

Knowledge: ....

Risk factor: ....

Action: ....

Chapter 6: Why your foot is a fortress.

Knowledge: ....

Risk factor: ....

Action: ....

Chapter 7: Foot structure and deformity.

Knowledge: ....

Risk factor: ....

Action: ....

Chapter 8: Healing rate.

Knowledge: ....

Risk factor: ....

Action: ....

Chapter 9: Circulation.

Knowledge: ....

Risk factor: ....

Action: ....

Chapter 10: Neuropathy – how is your dashboard?

Knowledge: ....

Risk factor: ....

Action: ....

Chapter 11: Infection.

Knowledge: ....

Risk factor: ....

Action: ....

Chapter 12: Be on guard.

Knowledge: ....

Risk factor: ....

Action: ....

Introduction to Part Three: Know where you stand.

Knowledge: ....

Risk factor: ....

Action: ....

Chapter 13: The foot MOT.

Knowledge: ....

Risk factor: ....

Action: ....

Chapter 14: Commit to yourself.

Knowledge: ....

Risk factor: ....

Action: ....

Chapter 15: Let your friends or family help.

Knowledge: ....

Risk factor: ....

Action: ....

Chapter 16: Commitment to a health professional.

Knowledge: ....

Risk factor: ....

Action: ....

Month 5.

Chapter 2: Are your feet killing you?

Knowledge: ....

Risk factor: ....

Action: ....

Chapter 3: Knowledge is power.

Knowledge: ....

Risk factor: ....

Action: ....

Chapter 4: Change your mindset, change your life.

Knowledge: ....

Risk factor: ....

Action: ....

Chapter 5: Time for action.

Knowledge: ....

Risk factor: ....

Action: ....

Chapter 6: Why your foot is a fortress.

Knowledge: ....

Risk factor: ....

Action: ....

Chapter 7: Foot structure and deformity.

Knowledge: ....

Risk factor: ....

Action: ....

Chapter 8: Healing rate.

Knowledge: ....

Risk factor: ....

Action: ....

Chapter 9: Circulation.

Knowledge: ....

Risk factor: ....

Action: ....

Chapter 10: Neuropathy – how is your dashboard?

Knowledge: ....

Risk factor: ....

Action: ....

Chapter 11: Infection.

Knowledge: ....

Risk factor: ....

Action: ....

Chapter 12: Be on guard.

Knowledge: ....

Risk factor: ....

Action: ....

Introduction to Part Three: Know where you stand.

Knowledge: ....

Risk factor: ....

Action: ....

Chapter 13: The foot MOT.

Knowledge: ....

Risk factor: ....

Action: ....

Chapter 14: Commit to yourself.

Knowledge: ....

Risk factor: ....

Action: ....

Chapter 15: Let your friends or family help.

Knowledge: ....

Risk factor: ....

Action: ....

Chapter 16: Commitment to a health professional.

Knowledge: ....

Risk factor: ....

Action: ....

Month 6.

Chapter 2: Are your feet killing you?

Knowledge: ....

Risk factor: ....

Action: ....

Chapter 3: Knowledge is power.

Knowledge: ....

Risk factor: ....

Action: ....

Chapter 4: Change your mindset, change your life.

Knowledge: ....

Risk factor: ....

Action: ....

Chapter 5: Time for action.

Knowledge: ....

Risk factor: ....

Action: ....

Chapter 6: Why your foot is a fortress.

Knowledge: ....

Risk factor: ....

Action: ....

Chapter 7: Foot structure and deformity.

Knowledge: ....

Risk factor: ....

Action: ....

Chapter 8: Healing rate.

Knowledge: ....

Risk factor: ....

Action: ....

Chapter 9: Circulation.

Knowledge: ....

Risk factor: ....

Action: ....

Chapter 10: Neuropathy – how is your dashboard?

Knowledge: ....

Risk factor: ....

Action: ....

Chapter 11: Infection.

Knowledge: ....

Risk factor: ....

Action: ....

Chapter 12: Be on guard.

Knowledge: ....

Risk factor: ....

Action: ....

Introduction to Part Three: Know where you stand.

Knowledge: ....

Risk factor: ....

Action: ....

Chapter 13: The foot MOT.

Knowledge: ....

Risk factor: ....

Action: ....

Chapter 14: Commit to yourself.

Knowledge: ....

Risk factor: ....

Action: ....

Chapter 15: Let your friends or family help.

Knowledge: ....

Risk factor: ....

Action: ....

Chapter 16: Commitment to a health professional.

Knowledge: ....

Risk factor: ....

Action: ....

Quick reference guide.

This quick reference guide gets straight to the point: what can you do to keep yourself safe and sound in the sweet spot?

It looks at the following groups:

1. People with pre diabetes.

2. Newly diagnosed:

   a. no complications.

   b. with complications.

3. Long-term diagnosed:

   a. no complications.

   b. with complications.

4. Understanding type 1 versus type 2 and gestational diabetes explained.

5. Living with a foot deformity.

6. To chop or not to chop. That is the question.

7. People with diabetes who have had an amputation.

In its broadest sense the diabetic sweet spot can be applied to blood glucose control because having optimal control will mean that you are at least risk of developing any of the complications those of us with diabetes potentially face.

This section will touch on how best to stay in the sweet spot from the point of view of good glucose control. This is relevant to anyone with diabetes be it type 1, type 2 or pre diabetes. I've broken the information down into sub-groups so that you can easily find the section that's most relevant to you. I hope you'll also make it your mission to help others who are at a different stage or may be presenting in a different way.

1. People with pre diabetes, at high risk of developing diabetes or someone who's worried because it runs in their family.

Pre diabetes, sometimes called borderline diabetes, is an increasing problem across the globe. Many of us will have family members or are ourselves pre diabetic without being aware of it.

Fewer still are aware of the implications of allowing it to develop into diabetes and what measures they can take to prevent it doing so.

You can think of pre diabetes as the very beginning of type 2. At this early stage you have the opportunity to sort yourself out and prevent full-blown type 2.

A person is said to have pre diabetes when there are higher than normal glucose levels in their blood, but that level is not high enough to classify them as diabetic.

In general,you will be told you have pre-diabetes if your fasting blood sugars have readings of 5.5 and 7.0 Mmol/L or if you have a Hba1c of 6-6.4% (42-47 Mmol/L). It is commonly associated with a poor diet and is often found in the western world where processed foods and excessive sugar, fat and salt and lower fibre content have become an increasingly large part of our staple diet.

If you or your loved one has pre diabetes it may be helpful to think of yourself as standing at a fork in the road of your life. You have a choice to turn one way to a better, more healthy life, or you can stay on the road you're used to.

It's an exciting choice but unfortunately one that isn't made by most people who continue to plod along in the same old rut. When driving on a long journey the main road is easier, it gets us there faster with fewer bumps and sharp turns. So too the path to a healthy lifestyle can seem daunting to someone who has become accustomed to the convenience of the unhealthy main road.

Yet just as country lanes are usually more beautiful and enjoyable to drive along, so too the healthy path will lead to much better experiences once you have chosen to travel along it.

The unhealthy highway will seem easier but don't get caught out because getting stuck in a motorway traffic jam is no fun. Living an unhealthy lifestyle will catch up with you eventually and often it is when pre diabetes tips over into diabetes.

The Longevity Lane approach may seem harder, and often it is at first, but it will become easier especially if you have support from your family. If not, a friend could help or you could join a sweet spot group, and perhaps you could join the forum at **www.undefeeted.org/forum**. Those difficult times will become less intense and less frequent as time goes by.

The unhealthy highway.	Longevity Lane
Processed food is often cheaper.	*Over time you'll develop a healthy appetite and so will eat less.*
It's easier to prepare.	*Get used to new ways of preparing food. Make double the amount and freeze or eat it the next day.*
Convenient.	
Readymade.	
Tasty (this is usually because our taste buds are already affected by all the processed food and have become less sensitive).	*Your taste buds get used to less salt or sugar. Over time processed food begins to taste wrong, even toxic.*
No bumps along the way, e.g. peer pressure.	*Difficult to eat properly.*
It's an effort to exercise.	*It gets easier and more enjoyable the more you do it.*
Exercise can cause injury.	*Be sensible and take it easy with a gradual approach.*
This road is easier – no discipline is required.	*Discipline is critical. Get someone to hold you accountable.*

You are also at a greater risk of having pre diabetes and subsequently diabetes if you:

- Are of Asian, Middle Eastern or Afro-Caribbean descent.
- Are overweight with a high body mass index.
- Have a large waist.
- Have a close family member such as a parent or sibling who has diabetes.
- Have high cholesterol.
- Have high blood pressure.

As pre diabetes is the precursor of diabetes the symptoms are similar although usually not so pronounced. They can include thirst, needing the toilet more, and feeling lethargic and sometimes feeling hungry even shortly after eating a meal, especially if it was high in carbohydrate.

If you have these symptoms go and see your doctor who can do some simple blood tests to check if you have pre diabetes. Remember: if it is a positive diagnosis **it will be easier to reverse at this stage**.

If someone with diabetes is reading this, don't skip it thinking it's irrelevant. Give some thought as to whether any of your friends or family members fit into the risk categories and are therefore likely to be joining you as someone with diabetes. You may be their only chance of turning their life around and avoiding the development of diabetes with all of its associated risks.

2. Newly diagnosed.

Broadly speaking people seem to fall into one of three categories at the time of their diagnosis.

- You are shocked and understand the need to do something about it.

- You go into denial and do nothing.

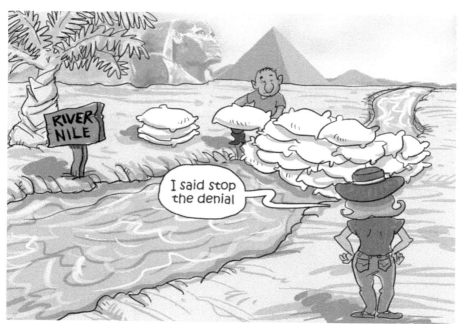

Let's face it... You're at risk... Now accept it!

- The vast majority seem to lie in-between and float in and out of the other two areas, the long-term result being that they become less and less aware of their need to control their blood sugars. This can continue for years until something like a retinopathy diagnosis or foot problem highlights to them once again the importance of being in control. Unfortunately by then it is often too late to make a big difference and the person is already set in their ways.

Furthermore as people can live with high blood sugars for years either as a person with pre diabetes or as an undiagnosed diabetic, deterioration behind the scenes may already be present albeit not severe enough for the symptoms to be recognised. So **at diagnosis you may already have complications**.

a. No complications.

The important thing here is to realise that you are at greater risk and that although you may not have any obvious symptoms there may be some lurking in the background. These can develop gradually and with no warning so that for example a person becomes much less resistant to infection.

In the case of someone like this it is important that they get into good habits from day one. They should get into the sweet spot recognising they have a lot to learn and they need to fully accept they are at risk (which will normally require an assessment from a podiatrist). They should then take appropriate action and, over time, adopt all the good habits while dropping the bad ones.

b. With complications.

If you have complications at diagnosis it is important not to give up, get depressed or live in denial. Embrace your condition and make it your mission to learn all you can, not just about diabetes but also about the specific effect it has had on your life. Even more important is to learn what you can do to best live with any problems you have. The second part of this book dealt specifically with the complications concerning the feet of people with diabetes and, crucially, how to prevent those problems getting worse.

The diabetic sweet spot process throughout this book should help you get into and remain in this safe haven. But as always the onus is on you to respond to what you read.

Online diabetic sweet spot groups have been set up for the sole purpose of helping people like you feel in control and not isolated by your condition. They are a platform for you to share struggles and victories and aim to provide an option for being held accountable. Eventually, I hope to see local sweet spot groups throughout the country, but until then the online resources at **www.undefeeted.org** can be your lifeline.

I also strongly encourage you to ask someone in your life to be your sweet spot buddy. They'll know your personal struggles and can share theirs so that together you can learn how to live in control of your diabetes.

3. Long-term diagnosed person with diabetes.

If you have had the diagnosis for a number of years, you may already have developed complications or be gradually starting to develop them. If you have lived to the best of your ability in the sweet spot by eating sensibly and exercising regularly then hopefully you will have maintained good blood sugars and so won't have developed any major problems. However there may be some deterioration that you are unaware of due to a combination of age and your diabetes.

a. No perceived complications.

It's great that you have managed your diabetes well so far but remember you need to remain vigilant as things can deteriorate slowly behind your back and then accelerate when you least expect it.

It's like parents who don't see their child's growth and progress as much as a grandparent who only sees them every few months – because they see their children every day parents can be blind to ongoing changes. Often people with diabetes don't notice the gradual increased severity of their condition or deterioration of their sensitivity or circulation or other aspects of their health. Don't get complacent. Treat yourself as you would a car; get a professional to give you the equivalent of an MOT once a year. This should show up any deterioration early allowing you to stay in the diabetic sweet spot.

b. **With complications.**

If you have had your diabetes a while and have either been told or you've become aware that you have problems then don't be too dismayed. Okay so you can't turn back the hands of time but you can do the next best thing which is to learn how to manage the problems with the least amount of risk of them deteriorating further. As the old saying goes 'a stitch in time saves nine'.

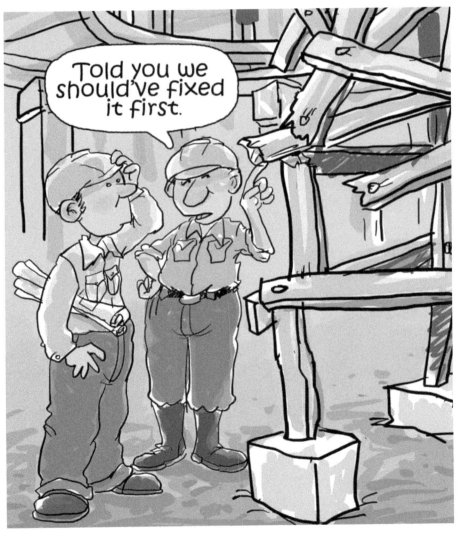

A stitch in time saves nine!

I would point out here that if you have become aware, for example of some numbness in your feet, that level of awareness is nowhere near deep enough. You need to be acutely aware of the dangers you face and the only way is to have a one-on-one assessment with a podiatrist who will tell you the degree of risk you are at and what to do about it. This book is a good resource but a personal professional assessment by an appropriate specialist is the best way to keep yourself safe as no book can specifically address your particular degree of deterioration or risk.

It's not ideal to have complications but at least you can manage them. Get into the diabetic sweet spot and make it your life's mission to take control of your condition and arrest any problems.

4. Understanding type 1 versus type 2 and gestational diabetes.

If I was given a pound every time someone told me they had the mild form of diabetes because they had type 2 and not type 1, I would be a very rich man. The public is misinformed about this issue and I even see the same dangerous misunderstanding on diabetes forums. I believe that we need to educate early on. Within the first year of her diagnosis my daughter had to sit through a school assembly where no differentiation was made between type 2 and her type 1. So all her friends and foes at school came out thinking she had become diabetic because of eating lots of sweets. That kind of message is harmful and simply not true, the cause of type 1 diabetes is not linked to a bad diet or being overweight.

Likewise many people think and often say that type 1 is the worst type to have. In some ways this is true but let me explain why type 2 can often be more devastating.

First let's have a look at type 1. This is sometimes referred to as juvenile diabetes because the majority of cases are diagnosed during childhood, although it can be diagnosed at any age (The Juvenile Diabetes Research Foundation, otherwise known as JDRF, do incredible work supporting people with type 1 not only in how to best live with it, but also crucially in funding research into better treatments and ultimately a cure).

Contrary to type 2, type 1 is an autoimmune disease which is thought to be caused by a genetic predisposition combined with an external or internal environmental trigger. The result is that the person's immune system attacks their own insulin producing cells (beta cells) in the pancreas. It is not fully understood what triggers this although it may be a virus that stimulates the autoimmune response leading to no insulin production.

The symptoms of diabetes such as thirst, tiredness, weight loss and going to the toilet more often, develop as more and more beta cells are killed off and the body is no longer able to control its blood sugar levels.

A person with type 1 diabetes therefore requires insulin several times a day to be able to regulate their blood sugar levels. Type 1 is also sometimes referred to as insulin dependent diabetes. It is important that if you suspect a person has developed type 1 that you take them to the doctor as soon as possible as delay in treatment can be fatal.

The immediate symptoms of type 1 diabetes are all linked to the fact that the blood sugar cannot be regulated and so has risen considerably.

Symptoms to look out for:

- Extreme thirst (linked to point three in this list): The body is trying to clear out all the extra sugar in the blood and does so by you peeing more frequently thus you also get thirstier.

- Extreme tiredness due to the lack of insulin circulating meaning the cells can't access the energy from the sugar.

- Increased urination.

- Having to get up in the night for the toilet.

- Unexplained weight loss. If the body can't use the circulating sugar it thinks there is not enough and so starts to break down its fat reserves converting it into more sugar.

- Skin infections and genital itching.

Type 2 on the other hand may have similar symptoms but not as extreme as in type 1. It is caused partly by the body not producing enough insulin and partly by the cells becoming ineffective at using the insulin that it has produced.

In the past type 2 was only really found in adults over 40 but now with poorer diet and more sedentary lives it is increasingly being found in young adults, teens and even in kids. Type 2 is far more prevalent than type 1 with approximately 90% of diabetics in this category.

If you have been diagnosed with type 2 diabetes, it is likely you will have been told of the importance of a good diet and a daily exercise regime. This may in itself be enough to bring your blood sugars down to a safe level without the need for you to take medication. However, sometimes, for many reasons including apathy, it may be that you do require medication and if the control deteriorates more then you may even be given insulin in addition to other treatment. Most medicines cause side effects so it's best to control your type 2 diabetes through lifestyle changes that keep you in the diabetic sweet spot. I would like to mention here two people I admire both at the forefront of helping with reversing type 2 diabetes.

Firstly, Professor Roy Taylor of Newcastle University famed for his intense low calorie diet that in affect mimics the effects of having a gastric band. The 8 week diet kickstarts the body's ability to use its insulin as well as helping the pancreas produce more insulin. For further information, check out **http://www.ncl.ac.uk/magres/research/diabetes/reversal.htm**

Secondly, Dr David Cavan, who is the Director of Policy and Programmes at the International Diabetes Federation. He has recently written a book entitled *Reverse your Diabetes* which is getting great reviews. Type 1 is not reversible although thanks to JDRF and others, we are getting closer to a cure and improving methods of controlling blood sugars.

> *In the past type 2 was only really found in adults over 40 but now...it is increasingly being found in young adults, teens and even in kids.*

For type 1 that will include the need for insulin and for type 2 it may include medication plus insulin. Whatever medication you need to take, the fact is that both type 1 and type 2 will benefit from a better diet and daily exercise.

People say type 1 is the worst because without injecting insulin several times a day the people who have this condition will die, whereas it is not uncommon for people with type 2 to live for five to 10 years with no immediate threat to their life and without any need for extra insulin.

In recent years technology has meant that people don't need to inject any longer, they can administer their insulin by means of a pump. Future exciting developments should make control much easier and hopefully one day we will find a cure.

Both types can lead to poor control of blood glucose which, when elevated over a long period of time, can cause the classic complications of diabetes: heart disease, stroke, retinopathy, kidney disease, neuropathy, and foot disease.

Because of its severity and the need for insulin, type 1 can often be controlled better than type 2 where control may rely upon balancing exercise and diet with some medication. So in fact a person with poor control over their type 2 diabetes may over time have higher blood glucose and its ensuing complications particularly with regards to the lower limbs.

I advise my clients that type 2 is not likely to kill you with one quick incident as type 1 can through extreme hypo or hyperglycaemia. **But it is more likely to be a silent killer** gradually eroding your health and setting up your body for the perfect storm which can lead to a slow death.

For both types take the advice of your doctor, consultant and podiatrist with regards to medication and ensure you do your utmost to stay in the sweet spot, learning as you go along new ways of staying safe within it.

Gestational diabetes.

This is usually a transient condition in a pregnant lady resolving itself when the baby has been born although she may be at greater risk of developing type 2 later in life.

During pregnancy the mother's hormones are constantly changing and from three months onwards certain hormones produced by the placenta resist insulin. At the same time the baby is growing and these two factors mean that the mother requires two to three times more insulin than before the pregnancy. In approximately one in 20 pregnancies[5] the mother is not

---

[5] The NHS puts the figure at 1 in 6 while Diabetes UK and the American Diabetes Association agree on 1 in 20.

able to make enough insulin. The blood sugars rise and the baby is said to have gestational diabetes.

Ladies at greatest risk of developing gestational diabetes are likely to have one of the following risk factors:

- They have a close relative who has had gestational diabetes or is now type 2.

- They have had gestational diabetes themselves.

- They are of Asian, Middle Eastern or Afro-Caribbean descent.

- They have a BMI greater than 30.

- They have previously had a baby that weighed more than 10lbs.

The symptoms for gestational diabetes are similar to type 2 namely: thirst, dry mouth, tiredness, having to urinate more often, and having infections such as thrush (a yeast infection).

Applying the principles of the sweet spot will be enough for most women to control their gestational diabetes (learning about their condition, recognising the risk they are at and then acting appropriately by increasing exercise and adapting their diet).

However if blood glucose control is not maintained well medication and even insulin may be required as high blood glucose can be fatal for the baby, for example if the mum develops ketoacidosis. This happens when there is not enough insulin and the body has to get its energy from burning fatty acids, a by-product of which is acidic ketone bodies. This can also happen in type 1 and 2.

The symptoms to look out for are:

- Dehydration and thirst.
- Vomiting.
- Breathing becoming deep and laboured.
- Becoming confused and disorientated.
- Loss of consciousness and even coma.

5. Diabetes and foot deformities

We've looked at the different types of diabetes so it is now relevant to mention how important foot deformities are. Most of the factors that put the foot at risk in a person with diabetes are ones that develop as a direct result of high blood sugars.

In the Traffic Light System explained in chapters 13 and 16, deformity is one of the risk factors that can be present many years before developing diabetes. Thus it is important for you to check your own feet and see a podiatrist for a thorough examination where they will be able to tell you if you already have a potentially risky deformity or are developing one.

Having a deformity can mean the difference between being in the moderate risk category or the high risk category. We can do things at a young age to slow down and prevent these deformities and it may even be that at an older age, early in your diagnosis with diabetes, that surgery is indicated whilst you are still relatively healthy and more likely to heal.

A foot deformity greatly increases your risk of trauma by pressure on prominent areas of the foot causing a wound which, being diabetic, is less likely to heal and more likely to get infected and lead to amputation and possible death. You can read more about this in Chapter 7.

6. To chop or not to chop. That is the question.

Sometimes unfortunately your foot may have deteriorated to the point that your diabetic foot team may advise you that an amputation is necessary. Although this book is all about preventing that happening, there are times when undergoing an amputation of part of the foot may mean you are left with a remaining portion of your foot which will heal easier than just trying to heal the original sore. Additionally a surgeon may decide to remove more of the foot than may seem necessary to you. This is usually because leaving a prominent place on the foot is more likely to cause future ulceration and a route for infection to cause more serious tissue loss.

Although usually as much of the foot or leg will be saved as possible, sometimes the amputation is carried out further up the leg simply because you will stand a better chance of healing up well and not re-ulcerating.

This can be a difficult thing to understand when faced with the dilemma A classic case I became aware of was a gentleman where four toes had been amputated leaving only the middle one. This, although looking better on paper as a less serious amputation than, for example, taking the front half of the foot away, is likely to cause future problems with further amputation being necessary. It is worth remembering that every time a person ulcerates, it has the potential to lead not only to infection and amputation, but also to death and so any surgery should aim to leave you with the best possible remaining portion of your limb to allow you to keep mobile with the least possible risk to that limb or indeed the other one.

Perhaps this can be likened to how firefighters sometimes prevent forest fires from spreading by creating a controlled fire to burn off any combustible materials so that when the raging forest fire arrives, it has nothing to fuel it and so puts itself out.

If ever you are in this position, then please discuss with your surgeon and team what they are planning and what your rehabilitation process will entail and what are the likely future risks you may be exposed to.

7. People with diabetes who have had an amputation.

Thankfully being diabetic doesn't mean you will inevitably have an amputation; it's just that you are more at risk of that fate.

However if you have already had the misfortune of undergoing one whether it be a toe, a partial foot or below knee, then you are at a greater risk statistically of either further amputation or even death.

There are several reasons for this which you should take into account. For you, getting back into the sweet spot is likely to require very specific knowledge, risk awareness and actions.

Having undergone an amputation, it is likely that your diabetes has developed to a stage where your lower limbs are already at risk. Indeed in the Traffic Light system just having had an amputation in the past automatically puts you in the red high risk category.

Once you have had the amputation the new wound has to heal so you will be given specific advice regarding things like the frequency of dressing it, how to offload the area and how to keep it dry.

When it's healed it is likely that you will need bespoke shoes to offload any new areas subjected to increased pressure.

Often the intact leg is favoured and so the increase in pressure can cause that foot to develop pressure sores, especially under areas of significant callus.

Remaining in the safety zone of the sweet spot will often entail you being given in-depth knowledge of the specific problems you are likely to encounter. It will mean you need to realise just how much more at risk you are and it will also mean you have to fall into line and actively start changing your lifestyle and habits for the better.

Examples of how your lifestyle may have to change will vary on an individual basis but may include:

- Having to attend a hospital clinic several times a week to ensure the wound heals.

- Resting the foot or leg to avoid the wound being subjected to further trauma.

- Not being able to work.

- Having to wear a cast or boot to offload any remaining areas of the foot which otherwise would be subjected to further trauma.

You may not be able to walk as you used to and yet you still need to keep active. You therefore may need to begin some upper body exercises to keep the blood pumping and to burn up those blood sugars.

You may not be able to wear conventional shoes and have to have special surgical shoes made. These are unlikely to be fashionable but they will keep you safely in the sweet spot.

One of the key attitudes for a person who has undergone an amputation is vigilance. Keeping an eye open for further problems either at the site of the amputation or elsewhere is absolutely vital.

One of the key attitudes for a person who has undergone an amputation is vigilance.

By itself though, this vigilance is useless unless you or your carer take action. Speed of implementation for this action is critical and any changes in either foot should be reported that day to the specialist diabetic foot protection team. You should have been given their contact details on being discharged from the hospital.

If your diabetes has become bad enough to have led to an amputation then not only are you likely to heal slower, be more at risk of infection, to have lost sensation and have peripheral vascular disease, but also you are more likely to have had changes in your eyes.

If you have developed retinopathy it's all very well me telling you to be vigilant but you may not even be able to see your feet. This is where having a friend, spouse or carer as a buddy can be essential as they can (and should) do daily checks of both of your feet. Again they should immediately report any deterioration to your foot protection team.

If you don't have anyone you can ask, then buy yourself a camera and take photos of your foot both on top and underneath by photographing the soles' reflection in a mirror leaning against the wall.

Better still get a selfie pole and use it and your phone to take a photo of the underside of your feet. Some of the better ones have a button on them that remotely takes the photo. You can then send it by email or whatsApp to a buddy, family member or friend who can alert you to any issues so that you can get help.

Undefeeted™ is also planning to offer a service assessing photos remotely, you can find out more about it at **www.undefeeted.org/footieselfie**.

Of course actually having a buddy inspect your feet in person is always better than someone looking at a photograph as they can check for such things as temperature, but a professional eye cast over a photo may well spot something of significance that the untrained eye could overlook. I suppose the best long distance option is having someone else take the photo and sending it, along with their observations, to a professional.

You will be able to do this via the Undefeeted™ app once it has been launched. Check out **www.undefeeted.org/footieselfie** and we will keep you updated on the launch date for this service.

Final Remarks

Feet aren't just "plates of meat".

Even today walking down the street in the east end of London, if you witnessed someone dropping something heavy on their toes you would be likely to hear, amongst other expletives, the words, "AAARGH MY PLATES OF MEAT!" The phrase "plates of meat" is cockney rhyming slang for the feet.

Recently I was in a supermarket with my 2 smallest children doing their best to drive me insane. We had already been in the store for a while and the trolley was full of all the things we needed for the week and, I suspected, some we didn't that had been smuggled in when Dad wasn't looking.

I had managed to dissuade the kids from the turkey twizzlers and other equally unhealthy sources of protein and had arrived back at the fresh meat area. This Sunday, we would have a nice piece of meat for a roast dinner.

I waited patiently at first as the couple in front of me spent what seemed like forever to choose the perfect shoulder of lamb whilst blocking everyone else with their trolley. But as my kids were trying to use the trolley as a go-kart, I became a little more agitated and muttered under my breath that it would soon be past its sell-by date.

Eventually they had their prized joint and vacated the area. As he walked off, I noticed the man had a bad limp and I wondered to myself what was wrong (as a podiatrist, I find myself watching the way people walk and doing mini diagnoses in my head). That day it struck me that he was probably like most people and had probably spent more time (and money) choosing the meat for one Sunday dinner than on looking after his feet throughout his whole lifetime.

My hope and prayer is that you, the reader, will no longer see your feet or treat them as merely lumps of meat on the end of your legs, but will have learned from this book how to treat them with the same, if not more, respect than your teeth, eyes and even your hair. Above all, remember you only get one pair of feet and diabetes should not be allowed to be the reason for them not remaining intact on the ends of your legs serving you well for the rest of your life. In conclusion then, the mission of Undefeeted™ above and beyond preventing avoidable diabetic amputations on a global scale is on a personal level to ensure you as an individual are able to continue doing the things you enjoy with those you love for the rest of your life.

Acknowledgements.

I would like to thank the following team of people who have worked tirelessly behind the scenes to get *Undefeeted by diabetes* into your hands.

On a professional level I would like to thank Dr David Armstrong, Duncan Stang, Gerry Rayman and Mike Edmonds for the gift of their time, their input and their encouragement and enthusiasm for the Undefeeted™ campaign.

Secondly to those colleagues of mine who have supported me and challenged me throughout my career and in particular to Peter Graham and Debbie Delves.

For Daniel Priestley for giving me the initial seed of an idea that a book would be a great thing to do.

To those who have helped in the production of the book, for Chris Day and his team at Filament you have been amazing.

To my editor/writing mentor /coach Jane Mallin for being a constant source of inspiration, for motivating me when I needed it, for whipping me into action when I was slacking, and for encouraging me for work well-written whilst not being afraid to speak her mind about substandard writing. Jane you are fantastic.

To James Lavers for his never-ending input and advice on the whole project.

To Johnny Fratto for helping give Undefeeted™ momentum with introductions to some amazing celebrities.

To my team at Circle Podiatry for your support when I have been consumed by the book and not been present in the practice.

For all the patients who have shown support for what we are doing.

Lastly but by no means least thank you to my family and friends for their support, giving me time-out to write and putting up with the grumps and especially for my wife Tina for always being a support and inspiration at the exact times I needed it most. Thank you to my daughter Jasmine whose bravery at her diagnosis was incredible and who shares with me a parallel journey with diabetes.

Finally Thank you to God for giving me the talent and ability to put these words together ,for blessing me abundantly in my journey of life so far, and for his word that is a constant source of inspiration for me.

About the author.

Peter Allton is the Clinical director of Circle Podiatry, the UK's only multi award winning podiatry brand. As a podiatrist his life's work has been fixing people's feet and lower limbs. He is also the founder of Undefeeted™ a global campaign powered by Circle Podiatry with the mission to reduce the number of avoidable diabetes-related lower limb amputations.

Initially spending 13 years working in community and hospital clinics for the NHS in the UK, Peter set up in private practice in 2001 founding Circle Podiatry. He qualified as a podiatrist in 1988 and has treated more than 200,000 feet.

In 2005 his wife Tina left her teaching career to become practice manager and has become a driving force behind the success of Circle Podiatry. Together they have led their team to win numerous awards and claim the title of being the UK's only multi award- winning private podiatry brand.

Peter has always been aware of the importance of diabetes when treating feet especially since he was diagnosed with type 2 in 2010. But it was his daughter's diagnosis with type 1 at the age of 11 that changed the emphasis of his career forever. He realised he was probably in the unique position of being the only podiatrist in the world with type 2 and a daughter with type 1 and he has since made it his mission to do something about the horrific diabetes statistics.

Every 20 seconds somewhere in the world a person with diabetes is undergoing a lower limb amputation. It is estimated that 85% of these could have been avoided. It is Peter's vision that over the next 10 years the Undefeeted™ campaign will help to cut that number to one every minute.

Peter can be contacted via **contact@undefeeted.org** and welcomes any helpful input, support and testimonials of your journey into the diabetic sweet spot.